Junk Food
Vegan

and How Not to Become One!

DAVID REAVELY

B.Ed (Hon), Cert Ed. D.N. Med mBANT CNHC

Published by: Monster Publishing Limited.

ISBN 978-1-9196064-4-6

Book Designed by Nonon Tech & Design

Also, by David Reavely

The Natural Athlete
(Diviniti Publishing)

The Cool Kid's Guide to Healthy Eating
(First and Best in Education)

**The Big Fat Mystery: How Hidden Food Intolerances Can
Sabotage Your Attempts to Lose Weight**
(Metro Books)

Healthy Eating and Pollution Protection for Kids: A Parent's Guide
(O Books)

The Beginners Guide to Rejuvenation
(Amazon e-book)

**Alternative Cancer Treatments:
The Essential Source of Self-Empowering Information**
(Amazon Books)

Hypothiocyanite: Nature's Answer to Infections
(A Practitioner's Guide)

About the author

David, a former teacher and now a nutritional therapist, is a member of the British Association for Nutrition and Lifestyle Medicine (BANT) and is registered with the Complimentary and Natural Healthcare Council (GNHC). He gained a diploma in nutritional medicine in 2006 after studying with the highly regarded Plaskett College of Nutritional Medicine, now merged with Thames Valley University in London, UK.

David has written articles on nutrition for Athletics Weekly Magazine and numerous other periodicals, and is a former host for the Holistic Health Show that was broadcast from Maidstone T.V. Studios in Kent, England.

His work has been supported over the years by world-renowned naturopath and prolific author, Jan de Vries, a former 'health guru' on the UK's 'Good Morning' Show.

He has appeared in the media on several occasions and his advice and opinion have been sought by BBC Radio Kent and South-East T.V. based in the UK

Disclaimer

This publication is designed to provide health educational data in regard to the subject covered. It is a reference and experiential work of general interest and benefit to readers and is not intended to treat, diagnose or prescribe. The information contained herein is in no way to be considered a substitute for consultation with a competent health care professional. If pregnant or breastfeeding, you should consult a qualified doctor or health practitioner before embarking on the application of nutritional advice in this book. Skilled medical opinion is advised on specific health complaints before any course of action is taken.

Endorsement

I agree with the premise of David's book. Even though white sugar and margarine are vegan, they are NOT healthy. Health comes from living in line with nature and our nature.

Any step you take in the direction of fresh, whole, raw, organic and more plant-based is a step in the direction of health. If you are vegan, remember to take a B12 supplement.

Udo Erasmus

Best-selling author of *'Fats that Heal Fats that Kill'*

Creator of world-renowned Udo's Choice oil

Table of Contents

Foreword

I strongly recommend reading this Junk Food Vegan Book by David Reavely.

The book is useful for anyone who is looking for a well written & reference book with factual information about a vegan diet.

The information in this book is so valuable for anyone looking for a Healthy Vegan Lifestyle. It has valuable information as well as recipes to help anyone to switch from the SAD diet that leads to chronic disease to the Healthy Vegan lifestyle to help you live to 111 +++ Years.

Professor Dr. George Grant, B.Sc. Hons., M.Sc., M.Ed., Ph.D., IMD, DHS
Former Senior Consultant for Health Canada, FDA & CDC
Best Selling Author of 20 books
Senior Editor of 12 Journals.
www.academyofwellness.com; www.your101ways.com

Prof. Dr. George Grant, Ph.D., Global Wellness Ambassador;
www.academyofwellness.com ♡
https://calendly.com/drwellness

Live to the fullest, Love unconditionally, Learn daily, Laugh always, Let Go and Leave a Legacy forever. Live the life you Love; Love the Life you Live. Live without Pretending/Love without Depending/Listen without Defending/Speak without Offending.

Introduction

There are lots of good reasons to adopt a vegan lifestyle. Namely, it doesn't involve killing animals, it's better for the environment and it can be better for our health. Moreover, there's no doubt that there's an increasing interest in adopting a vegan diet and dare I say it? It's becoming quite trendy. In fact, I can see certain parallels between this development and the growth of the gluten-free industry. Unfortunately, that's where the problem lies.

First of all, let me say that as a nutritional therapist with a special interest in the effects of food intolerances on human health, I'd be the first to agree that gluten sensitivity, whether in the form of an allergy or intolerance (they are different but can be equally damaging to the body) needs to be taken seriously and thankfully more people are aware that it is a real condition. Having said this, what happened in the wake of such increasing awareness is that the food manufacturing companies recognised a gap in the market and began churning out all of these gluten-free products that are very unhealthy. This is because the vast majority of these products are made from refined grains (albeit those not containing gluten), additives, sugar and unhealthy fats. This is a key observation, because all of the scientific evidence that we have at our disposal points towards processed foods being a major factor in the causation of **DISEASE!**

When people ask me what the problem is when it comes to vegan friendly foods, I tell them it's the same thing. The food manufacturers are seizing the opportunity to meet the increasing demand for vegan friendly food products and just like those unhealthy gluten-free foods that have flooded the market, we now have a tsunami of mostly processed vegan foods. Not all of them are unhealthy but having regularly scrutinised what is on offer, I can safely say that many of them are.

Now don't get me wrong; I'm not saying that a vegan junk food diet is as bad as the so-called SAD diet (standard American diet) which is now similar to the Western style of diet so prevalent in developed countries. The Americans, like the Brits consume lots of animal products along with all of the bad stuff we've already mentioned. Anyone who has read **The China Study** (T. Colin Campbell, PhD and Thomas M, Campbell II, MD, Benbella Books) which is based upon the largest study of human nutrition ever conducted, will surely conclude that animal products are a major factor in the causation of many of the chronic diseases that shorten the lives of millions of people every year. However, let me be brutally honest here, when I scrutinise the vegan food products that are on sale in health food shops and supermarkets in the UK and other countries, I'm acutely aware that the ingredients that make up these products are not conducive towards good health. Put simply, it's worth noting the following:

- They're lacking in nutrients
- They often consist of refined ingredients such as processed grains (e.g. rice flour, cornflour, wheat flour – few if any are whole grains)
- They often contain refined sugars including sucrose along with other sugars such as maltose and modified corn syrup
- They rely too much on processed soya, including genetically modified soya (unless it says GM free)
- They often contain artificial additives such as flavourings and preservatives
- Many contain unhealthy fats such as sunflower oil that have been subjected to heat. Sunflower oil is a polyunsaturated oil and is easily damaged by heat
- Some contain too much salt

Now here's the key point! If the aforementioned vegan friendly foods were to be eaten in limited amounts with the rest of the diet consisting of lots of fresh fruits and vegetables, with the addition of whole grains, nuts, seeds and pulses; then this wouldn't be perfect, but it would be much better than adhering to a diet that comprised predominately of the refined stuff. Unfortunately, I come across a lot of vegans who have come to rely on these vegan processed foods and as a consequence wonder why they become ill. In fact, thanks to my occupation, I encounter vegans who are suffering from heart complaints, hypertension, thyroid issues, arthritis, skin conditions, low energy, digestive issues and much more. The irony is that it's the commonly held belief amongst vegans that a so-called plant-based diet is naturally healthy.

Admittedly, several studies have shown that vegetarians and vegans tend to live longer and have less heart disease, strokes, cancer and other chronic diseases. Generally speaking, this does appear to be true, but **only if the diet is based upon a diet of whole foods.**

Having said this, it's worth remembering that it's the fruits and vegetables that should form the core of the diet, with the other whole foods eaten in lesser amounts. What's more, it's also worth remembering that grains do not suit everyone, and there is evidence that when it comes to people achieving a good standard of health, grains are counterproductive for some.

There are a number of books that address this subject, including Dr David Perlmutter's book, **Grain Brain: The Surprising Truth about Wheat, Carbs and Sugar – Your Brain's Silent Killers; Yellow Kite**, 16th Jan. 2014

Plant-Based or Vegan: Are they the same?

I often get asked this question as it's quite confusing for a lot of people. My own view is that the term plant-based doesn't necessarily mean adhering to a vegan diet. For example, if we analyse the diets of people from around the world who have a reputation for living a long and active life, with low incidence of chronic disease, we soon begin to realise that the thing they have most in common is that they live on a diet that is rich in plants in the form of fruits, vegetables and wholefoods. In the majority of cases, they have a small amount of animal produce in their diet.

Therefore, a whole -foods plant- based diet isn't the same as a vegan whole foods diet, as the latter doesn't include any animal produce.

CHAPTER 1
Is Eating Processed Vegan Foods Good for our Health?

So, when it comes to vegan food options, I'm not saying that they're all unhealthy as some are made using natural, whole food ingredients. For example, ice-cream made from coconut cream and sweetened with fruits. However, what kind of processed foods am I referring to? Well, here are some examples of products that are often manufactured using unhealthy ingredients:

1. Meat substitutes such as fake versions of the following: chicken, bacon, beef (e.g., minced beef), fish, etc.

2. Cheese and other dairy substitutes – usually a combination of coconut oil, flavourings (some of these are artificial), starch of some sort (e.g. maize starch), salt and other possible additives

3. Egg replacement powders

4. Vegan versions of mayonnaise and cooking sauces

5. Vegan ice-cream – often made with soya milk or coconut milk and usually packed with sucrose, glucose or other refined sugars. There are some that use nuts, such as cashew to create a delicious ice-cream alternative, and these are available in some supermarkets and health food shops. The ones to opt for are sweetened with more natural sweeteners such as date syrup, or better still, just fruits.

6. Vegan desserts such as chocolate mousse, custard, etc. – again, they usually contain a lot of refined sugars, except for a few; for example, one brand I spotted that contained only coconut sugar and fruit as a sweetener.

7. Vegan friendly breads and pastries (including the increasing number becoming available in fast food chains) – most that are on sale in supermarkets and some health food stores are made with refined carbs and other nutrient poor ingredients.

Let's Get Ingredient Savvy!

These are the types of ingredients that are used to manufacture a typical meat substitute:

Rehydrated textured soya protein, salt, sugar, yeast extract, sunflower oil, water, rapeseed oil and methyl cellulose

A typical vegan-friendly cake will often be based upon refined ingredients such as:

Chocolate 34% (cocoa solids 55%, Cocoa mass, sugar, cocoa butter, vanilla), flour (rice, tapioca, corn), palm oil, rapeseed oil, water, salt, natural colours, sugar, raisins, golden syrup, soya lecithin

Again, just to emphasise the point, these ingredients represent a health risk, especially when they are eaten at the expense of much healthier fruits and vegetables.

What About Coconut Oil?

Whether it's a good idea to consume coconut cream and coconut oil on a regular basis divides opinion; largely due to its saturated fat content. However, it's worth noting that the saturated fats in coconut oil are different from those found in animal fats such as butter. They contain medium chain triglycerides, which are thought to be handled differently by the body and are more easily broken down. Nevertheless, when it comes to consuming coconut oil, I think that we need to exercise caution as none of its purported health benefits are backed by research and some studies have shown that it does raise LDL ('bad' cholesterol), a cardiovascular risk factor. It's also likely that the coconut oils used in many of the vegan products on the market have been refined in contrast to those that are cold pressed and organic.

So, am I saying that vegans should be avoiding the consumption of coconut oil entirely? No, but I would definitely opt for cold-pressed coconut oil and coconut cream and use them only occasionally, whilst at the same time placing more emphasis upon using cold pressed oils that supply omega 3 and 6 essential fats, since these are the only ones that the body needs for health (see also Chapter 10, Key Nutrients for Vegans).

Is Processed Soya a Bad Thing?

US nutritionist Kaayla T Daniel who has studied the history of soya consumption, argues that the soya eaten in China and Japan, such as tofu and miso, is very different from the industrially processed variety used in today's Western food.

Daniel states that the soya bean originated in China, and according to her, the ancient Chinese called it 'the yellow jewel' and used it as 'green manure' to enrich the soil for growing other crops. Apparently, it didn't become a part of the staple Chinese diet until the Chinese developed a fermentation process that converted the bean into a paste, best known by its Japanese name, **miso**. The liquid that is poured off during this production is known as **soya sauce**. Daniel claims that the production of fermented products like tofu or tempeh destroys some of the alleged toxic compounds such as phytic acid, that occur naturally in soya, unlike modern factory methods used today.

In my opinion, this doesn't mean that all processed soya products are bad, especially if they're of the fermented variety and GM free; however, in my experience, keeping processed foods to a minimum whilst ensuring that vegetables and fruits form the core of the diet, along with other whole foods is the best way of promoting good health. In fact, I've witnessed this time and time again with clients who achieve a much better state of health after switching from eating processed foods to a more natural diet. They soon realise that there's no magic formula that is going to cure them of their ills; however, when you provide the right conditions for your body, its innate healing abilities are galvanised and healing will often take place.

Therefore, the message for vegans is clear:

Reduce or eliminate processed foods such as refined grains (wheat flour, white rice and pasta) and instead consume whole grains, fruits and vegetables, raw nuts, seeds and other whole foods. By adopting this way of eating you will undoubtedly benefit in the following ways:

- You will increase your intake of vital nutrients including vitamins, minerals and healthy fats that serve to help your body and mind to function at an optimal level
- You will decrease your intake of toxins and help your body to eliminate them from your tissues
- You will increase your intake of fibre which helps keep your digestive system working efficiently, as well as provide a favourable environment for the healthy bacteria that reside in your gut
- You will increase your resistance to disease
- You will help your body to overcome diseases that may already exist
- You will increase the likelihood of a lifespan that allows you to be physically active for longer

Key Principles!

If soya products agree with you, they can be included in your diet, but try to avoid becoming too dependent upon them. Moreover, you might wish to opt for products that are GM free wherever possible. Remember that unless you opt for GM free organic soya, or products made from such, you'll be ingesting traces of pesticides, fungicides, etc that have been used in the growing and storage process.

Also, it's worth noting that some manufacturers of vegan friendly foods are beginning to introduce alternatives to soya, using the likes of **pea protein** and **fava beans** instead. In fact, I purchased such a product from my local supermarket recently and was pleased to see that they had used mostly natural ingredients. So please do look out for these types of products.

What About Sugar?

Avoid eating too much sugar, especially refined table sugar (sucrose), including table sugar in its raw form, such as Muscovado (it's less refined and contains more minerals, but excessive consumption is also not conducive towards good health). Be wary of other sugars added to foods such as maltose, high fructose corn syrup, glucose and dextrose. From a health perspective, honey in small amounts is probably one of the healthiest forms of sugar; however, this doesn't sit well with strict vegans who regard its production as having to exploit bees. If you think that sugar substitutes are the answer, then you might have to think again! Artificial sugars such as aspartame and sucralose have been shown to cause adverse effects in some people.

Stevia in its natural whole leaf form is the only sugar substitute that I'd contemplate using. It has a slight after taste that some people don't like, but personally, it doesn't bother me. Try it and see what you think. I notice that a few different brands that produce whole leaf stevia are available on Amazon.

Why Sugar is Bad for Us!

- It's devoid of nutrients
- It's sometimes referred to as an anti-nutrient since it uses up some of the body's supply of nutrients in order to digest it. For example, did you know that refined sugar depletes B vitamins in the body?

- It causes tooth decay
- It disrupts blood sugar levels and excessive use has been implicated with increasing your risk of developing type 2 diabetes.
- It's a potent factor in the premature ageing of the skin
- It feeds infection
- It's one of the most addictive substances on earth, and boy, don't the food manufacturers know it!
- The body converts any excess into fat; therefore, it can be a significant factor in the cause of obesity.
- Sugar can increase the risk of coronary heart disease.
- It can promote the elevation of harmful cholesterol.
- Sugar can lead to chromium and copper deficiency.
- Sugar interferes with the absorption of calcium and magnesium – two key anti-ageing minerals.
- It's acid-forming
- Sugar affects cognition in children: According to a study that was published in the American Journal of Preventative Medicine, poorer childhood cognition occurred, especially in memory and learning, when pregnant women or their children consumed greater quantities of sugar. However, children's fruit consumption had beneficial effects and was associated with higher cognitive scores according to the researchers*

* "Associations of Prenatal and Child Sugar Intake with Child Cognition," by Juliana F.W. Cohen, ScD, Sheryl L. Rifas-Shiman, MPH, Jessica Young, PhD, and Emily Oken, MPH, MD.

- Sugar Causes Stress: When we're under stress, our bodies immediately kick into fight-or-flight mode, releasing large amounts of hormones. Moreover, the body has the same chemical response when blood sugar is low. After you eat a sweet snack, stress hormones begin to compensate for the crash by raising your blood sugar. This may lead to anxiety, irritability and feeling shaky.

Sugar and Ageing

Put simply, excess sugar in the blood accelerates ageing **big time!** This is because the glucose molecules react with proteins; this process is called **glycation**. Glycation is when sugar and proteins accumulate in muscles, joints and the skin. As crazy as it sounds, it's almost as if the tissues concerned become caramalised. This happens because the sugar-protein bonds make our collagen rigid. Collagen is a protein that acts like the body's intercellular 'scaffolding'. Not only do the tissues become rigid, communication between the cells that make up those tissues is interrupted. When glycation occurs in our arteries, it can cause them to harden. If it manifests itself in the collagen present in our skin, it can result in a lack of elasticity and wrinkling. Healthy skin is made up of collagen that is made of several layers that maintain the skin's elastic qualities. When glycation occurs, it's a bit like pouring superglue into the collagen matrix; the result is prematurely aged skin.

What's even worse is the fact that products produced as a result of glycation, known as **advanced glycation end products** (appropriately abbreviated to AGE's), tend to accumulate as we get older and may be implicated in a number of diseases, including Alzheimer's disease, atherosclerosis, diabetes and cataracts. Also, the protein-sugar combination increases the chance of the formation of blood clots.

CHAPTER 2
Some Healthy Vegan Substitutes

If you think that by switching to a vegan diet means that you'll be deprived of your favourite foods, then think again because there are a number of substitutes that you can use in order to make tasty alternatives.

I have included some of the key alternatives below:

Nutritional Yeast

This is a deactivated form of yeast that is a Godsend for people who find it difficult to give up cheese, because it really does taste like cheese. In fact, you can use it to make "cheese" sauces, macaroni cheese and even vegan Parmesan.

It's often stocked in health food stores and can also be bought on Amazon

Black Salt

Like Himalayan pink salt, black salt is mined from the Himalayas. I first came across it at a health show in London where I tasted it for the first time. An Asian lady gave me a tiny sample to try after telling me about how it tasted just like eggs due to its high sulphur content. To be honest, I thought she was exaggerating (or maybe eggaggerating!) until I placed a tiny amount on my tongue. I was amazed! It tasted just like eggs and I remember thinking that this condiment is going to be a key part of my diet. I have since discovered that you can mix it with avocados to make a vegan version of "scrambled eggs". Just mash the avocado with a little of the black salt.

You can buy this salt on Amazon and some health food stores, but do remember to look for the unrefined version and not one that is heat treated.

Coconut Oil

As already mentioned, coconut oil and cream feature in a lot of vegan products; for example, the oil is often used by vegans as a substitute for butter, since it has a similar texture. It's also used for baking, stir-fries, adding flavour and creaminess to home-made soups, nearly every vegan cheese you come across, and even for making desserts such as chocolate mousse. However, to reiterate my earlier advice, I would limit your consumption and place more emphasis upon sources of omega 3 and 6 essential fats whenever possible.

Ice-cream – Vegan Style

Simply freeze some bananas overnight, then blend them in a blender to make a delicious ice-cream. This is so simple and yet, because of the natural sweetness of the bananas along with their creamy texture, it really tastes like ice-cream. If you don't like bananas, try using frozen mango or similar tropical fruit.

You can also experiment by adding other flavours, such as a little coconut cream (or substitute avocado), natural vanilla essence and raw cacao powder.

This is a great alternative to many of the vegan ice-creams sold in supermarkets. Most of these are packed with refined sugars and artificial ingredients.

Home-Made Vegan Dessert

A quick method of making your own healthy vegan mousse is to purchase some diced frozen mango and place your chosen quantity in a blender, add 1 diced avocado, some coconut water, add an ingredient to add extra flavour (e.g., raw cacao powder); leave for 15 minutes to allow the frozen mango to soften and then whisk. The result is a delicious mousse that is naturally sweetened and contains no nasty additives.

Vegan Cream

You can replace dairy cream with full-fat coconut cream; or if you want to reduce calories you can opt for the reduced fat version.

It's excellent for making creamy home-made soups, curries, sauces and desserts.

Nut Butters

Nut butters are very versatile and can be used as a spread on toast, added to smoothies, desserts and even as an ingredient in salad dressings. You can also use them on pancakes; for example, pancakes made with almond flour as an alternative to wheat.

Top Tip!

The healthiest versions of nut butters are made from raw pressed nuts in contrast to the roasted varieties. If nuts are subjected to heat the volatile essential fats are damaged; for example, the Omega 3 essential fats found in walnuts and pecans. Consuming damaged fats is toxic for your cells, increasing the need for vitamin E and other antioxidants.

The same rule applies when purchasing seed butters such as pumpkin, sesame (tahini) and sunflower: avoid the ones that are roasted: **Raw is best!**

There are lots of varieties of raw nut butters available, including almond, walnut and pistachio. Alternatively, you can make your own using a peanut butter making machine that can also be used to make other nut butters

Bean Burgers

Beans can be a good alternative to meat and unlike meat they don't contain cholesterol or saturated fat.

All you have to do is to select a bean that you like, for example haricot, and after cooking them until they're soft, mix them with some shredded vegetables (carrot and cabbage for example), add some cooked garlic, onion and a binding ingredient such as a little brown rice flour and shape them into a burger. All that's left to do is to either lightly fry your vegan burger in extra virgin olive oil or coconut oil, or grill in the oven until golden brown.

Agar-Agar

If you are struggling to find a replacement for gelatine, Agar-agar is your answer. It's a natural gelling agent made from seaweed; however, it is colourless and tasteless. Use it to make desserts such as Panna Cota, jams and jellies.

It usually comes in the form of powder or flakes and once dissolved in water it will set just like gelatine, but a little firmer.

Cashew Nuts

Cashew nuts are a great everyday staple in your kitchen. They're very versatile and when soaked for a few hours and then blended with nutritional yeast, they can be used to make vegan cream cheese, various desserts, and as a cheese topping for cauliflower cheese. Creamed cashew nuts are also sometimes used as a base for vegan ice-cream.

If you have a de-hydrator you can also make your own spiced nuts. Simply soak the cashews and mix them with seasoning of your choice (example, black pepper and sea salt). Then place them in your de-hydrator for 24 hours. You can also use other pre-soaked nuts such as Brazil nuts, walnuts, pecans, pistachios and hazelnuts. Always opt for raw unsalted nuts. The low heat produced by the de-hydrator does not damage the healthy fats.

CHAPTER 3

How a Vegan Diet Can Promote Health

When it comes to restoring the health of the body, we need to remember that we are essentially a self-healing organism. The body has its own innate healing ability, and given the right conditions it will always strive to achieve a state of homeostasis, or balance. The reason why this balance is disturbed in the first place is usually due to years of eating processed, unnatural foods. Such foods are not only lacking in essential nutrients such as vitamins, minerals and 'live' enzymes, they often increase the level of toxins in the body. The combination of a lack of nutrients, nutritional imbalance and a high toxic load can often be tolerated for a number of years when we are young. However, more often than not, the end result is disease and premature ageing. Most holistic minded practitioners subscribe to the view that a toxic body will often lead to a diseased body; summed up in the following simple equation:

TOXICITY + LACK OF NUTRIENTS AND/OR NUTRITIONAL IMBALANCE = DISEASE

Bearing this in mind, it follows that in order to reverse or prevent a disease condition, we must provide the body with the right conditions to enable it to right itself. This is achieved when we make the necessary dietary and lifestyle changes; hence the rationale behind the following simple equation:

Detoxification + Balanced Plant-Based Diet + Correction of Nutritional Deficiencies = Self-Healing

Of course, there are other factors that can play their part in in any disease-forming process. These may include the following:

- A weakened immune system
- Excessive and prolonged stress

- Under-functioning eliminatory organs; for example, the colon and kidneys
- Over-stimulation due to excessive consumption of stimulants such as sugar, nicotine and caffeine.
- Over-consumption of food

Generally speaking, these factors can be corrected and in addition to adopting sensible eating habits, the body's innate healing abilities can be activated.

Vegans Take Note!

As far as the diet is concerned, the most important thing to remember is that the human body was meant to function on natural plant-based foods, in stark contrast to the 'foodless foods' that feature in the so-called Western style of diet so predominant in today's society. Many canned and packaged foods are devoid of important vitamins, minerals and enzymes. Not only do they lack these nutrients, your body uses up its own resources in order to digest them.

Getting the Balance Right

When it comes to the vegan diet, in aspiring towards achieving an optimum state of health, we must not only focus our attention on adhering to a natural diet; we also need to make sure we achieve the correct **acid/alkaline balance**. In health, our blood should have a pH of around 7.4, which is slightly alkaline. This is achieved quite easily when we base our diet on mostly alkaline-forming foods such as the majority of fruits and vegetables. However, the problem arises when we eat too many acid-forming foods. These make our bodies too acidic and upset the acid/alkaline balance. When this happens, our immune system becomes weaker, making us more prone to infections and other illnesses. We also become more susceptible to allergies and intolerances as well as osteoporosis (weakening of the bones). The latter condition arises because the body extracts alkalising minerals from the skeleton in an attempt to neutralise the acidity of the blood and tissues. In this way minerals such as magnesium and calcium are leached from the bones resulting in osteoporosis. This is why I feel that diets such as the Atkins Diet can be detrimental to health, because it is high in animal proteins which are very acid-forming.

In order to achieve a good pH balance, you need to remember the **80:20 rule**; this equates to a diet that comprises of 80% fruits and vegetables and 20% acid-forming foods such as pulses, soya (in its variety of forms), most grains, and most nuts and seeds.

Understandably, some people might find it difficult to imagine how the 80:20 rule would apply to their own eating habits. To get a rough idea, just imagine the food on your dinner plate comprising of approximately ¾ vegetables (alkaline-forming) and the remaining ¼ comprising of foods such as tofu, whole grains (example, quinoa or brown rice) and pulses. If you can apply that principle to most of your meals then you will be creating an alkaline blood system, which is conducive towards optimum health.

The Benefits of Raw and Living Foods

The principles encompassed within this book are based upon a diet that comprises of an abundance of raw vegetables with the addition of so-called living foods. Living foods are chlorophyll and enzyme rich raw plant foods. They comprise of the likes of sprouted seeds (e.g., alfalfa), fruits, vegetables, salad leaves and herbs. I would also include certain freshly-made juices, especially so-called green juices made with the likes of celery, cabbage, cucumber, spinach, kale and watercress. Wheatgrass juice is a particularly powerful healing juice and often forms the basis of healing programmes. The high chlorophyll content of such green drinks helps to detoxify the body, oxygenate the blood, whilst helping to rejuvenate the cells. They contain an abundance of vitamins, minerals and a wide range of helpful natural plant compounds that provide the body with greater protection from disease and promote vibrant good health.

In addition to sprouting seeds, you can also sprout nuts, pulses and grains. These sprouted foods are very rich in vitamins, minerals, amino acids and live enzymes. If you don't feel that you've got the time or inclination to sprout your own seeds, you do have the option of buying ready sprouted seeds that are available in many health stores and now in most supermarkets. You can also order the likes of ready sprouted sunflower and radish seeds from companies that specialise in this kind of thing.

(See also chapter 4 The Wonderful World of Sprouts!)

Another food group I would recommend is sea-greens, which includes seaweeds, such as kelp, wakame and nori. These are rich in trace minerals and iodine, which some people may be short of in their diets. I would suggest that you try to source sea-greens from areas that are relatively free from pollution, such as Norway. Personally, I would avoid produce from Japan and the surrounding areas due to possible radioactive contamination in the wake of the Fukishima accident. Maybe some parts of Japan are relatively free of contamination; however, I'm erring on the side of caution here.

What to Eat Vegan Check-list

A healthy vegan diet should revolve around the following vegetables:

Salad Greens	Sprouts	Vegetables
Spinach	Alfalfa	Asparagus
Kale	Adzuki beans	Broccoli
Chard	Broccoli	Cabbage
Dandelion greens	Fenugreek	Cauliflower
Lettuces	Pea greens	Celery

Scallions	Mustard	Green beans
Bok choy	Radish	Bell peppers
Watercress	Mung bean	Cucumbers
Sunflower greens	Chickpeas	Courgettes (zucchini)
Turnip greens	Cress	Squashes
Savoy cabbage		

Roots and Tubers	Sea Vegetables	Herbs (fresh)
Beetroot	Arame	Basil
Carrots	Dulse	Chives
Radishes	Kelp	Fennel
Garlic	Nori	Mint
Ginger	Wakame	Oregano
Onions		Parsely
Leeks		Rosemary
Garlic		Sage
Turnips		Tarragon
Sweet potatoes		Thyme
Swede		
Yams		

Fruits

The principle that underpins a healthy vegan diet is to base the majority of your diet upon vegetables with the addition of around 15 -20 % fresh fruits. Dried fruits such as raisins, dates, apricots and figs can be eaten sparingly.

The best fruits include the following:

Apples	Berries	Apricots
Pears	Melons	Oranges

Bananas	Grapefruit	Dates
Grapes (red and white)	Avocado *	Dried fruits
Cherries	Pineapple	Peaches
Kiwi	Starfruit	Plums
Watermelon		

*Avocados are a great source of healthy fats, but eat them in moderation, since too much fat will lower energy levels and slow down the healing process.

Seeds

Choose from pumpkin, sunflower, chia, hemp (shelled) and sesame. As mentioned in the foregoing, they should be eaten in their raw state, and not roasted and/or salted. You can also sprout them, which increases their digestibility and nutritional value.

Nuts

Choose from almonds, Brazil nuts, coconuts, filberts, pecans and walnuts. Again, eat them raw after soaking for at least six hours; or ideally in sprouted form.

Legumes

Grains, seeds and beans contain natural compounds that act as enzyme inhibitors to preserve them until the right growing conditions initiate them to begin sprouting. Therefore, if these foods are eaten without being soaked or sprouted, the enzyme inhibitors may interfere with their digestion and absorption of the nutrients that they contain. This is why some people find them difficult to tolerate.

Legumes (peas and beans) are a valuable source of fibre, minerals, carbohydrates and proteins. You can sprout the likes of aduki beans, chick-peas, mung beans and lentils. Whilst the bulk of your diet should comprise of low starchy vegetables; legumes are a valuable addition, but use them in moderation.

Grains

If grains are included in your diet, it's best to avoid all refined grains and their products, such as white rice and white wheat flour. The best grains include whole grain rice (all varieties, e.g. whole grain basmati, wild rice); quinoa, millet, buckwheat, rye and corn. Wheat isn't always tolerated well by everyone; however, if you don't appear to have a problem with wheat, I recommend that you opt for organically-grown whole grain varieties, including spelt, which is naturally lower in gluten. Ideally, grains should be sprouted and you can now buy some products in health food shops that are made from sprouted grains, such as different kinds of bread, some cakes and even crackers.

Juicing

Juicing can be a great addition to the diet because freshly made juices are rich in nutrients and live enzymes. Furthermore, green juices are high in chlorophyll, which is thought to play a key role in the healing process.

Although freshly made fruit juices do have some value as they're a valuable source of antioxidants and nutrients, they are also high in sugars, which will result in blood sugar peaks. The best solution is to consume mainly so-called green juices, whilst keeping the fruit juices to a minimum. It's also worth remembering that fruit juices such as apple, pineapple, pear and orange, should be diluted 50:50 with pure water (not tap water, unless filtered using a good quality filter).

A good example of a green juice would be the following:

2 sticks of celery, 1/2 of a cucumber, 2 handfuls of spinach, 1 apple or carrot (for sweetness), 1/4 of an unwaxed lemon and a small piece of fresh ginger (optional).

Other greens can be used instead of the spinach; for example, kale, green cabbage and lettuce. In fact, it's a good idea to vary which greens that you use in your juices in order to provide a wider range of nutrients.

Wheat Grass Juice

Wheat grass juice is known to be one of the most powerful cleansing juices, It's also one of the most therapeutic. This is why wheat grass juice is often included in detox programmes as well as being utilised in detox retreats and other similar establishments.

Aside from its ability to eradicate toxins, wheat grass juice is one of the richest sources of vitamins A and C in addition to a wide range of minerals, including cobalt, iron, magnesium, phosphorous, potassium, sodium, sulphur and zinc. It also contains all the essential amino acids, making it a complete protein. In addition, it's also rich in B vitamins, especially B17, otherwise known as laetrile which has a reputation for destroying cancer cells.

Wheat grass is also known to contain a very high amount of chlorophyll, the natural substance that gives plants their green colour. Chlorophyll has been shown to enhance the blood's capacity to carry oxygen to every cell of the body.

Dr. G.H. Erp-Thomas, a scientist with a specialism in soil composition, isolated more than one hundred elements from fresh wheat grass, after which he reached the conclusion that it is a complete food.

To learn more about the incredible benefits of wheat grass, I suggest that you purchase **The Wheat Grass Book** by Anne Wigmore, who purports to have used wheat grass juice to cure herself of cancer. Her early pioneering research into its benefits resulted in wheat grass being used as one of the cornerstones of the Life Change program at the Hippocrates Health Institute in Florida

Broccoli Sprout Juice!

This juice is extracted from broccoli sprouts which are produced from broccoli seeds that have sprouted.

This juice is an exceptional source of the antioxidant, sulforophane, a compound that's commonly found in cruciferous vegetables such as cabbage, broccoli and Brussels sprouts. Although broccoli itself is a good source, we find that the sprouts contain between 20-50 times more sulforophane than the parent plant. It's not surprising, therefore, that the juice extracted from broccoli sprouts may exert a powerful therapeutic effect.

Benefits

Sulforophane has been shown to have significant beneficial effects on our cells, including acting as a 'signaling' molecule that instructs the body to make more of the antioxidants, catalase, superoxide dismutase (SOD) and glutathione. These antioxidants are enormously protective in terms of neutralising the cell-damaging free radicals that are known to cause disease.

In addition to its antioxidant boosting effects, sulforophane has also been linked with the improvement of behaviours associated with autism spectrum disorder (ASD). One study in particular, involved 26 participants who received a daily dose of sulforophane. After 18 weeks of treatment improvements were noted in factors that included hyperactivity, irritability, lethargy communication and motivation.

This report was published online in **PNAS Early Edition**. PNAS is one of the world's most-cited and comprehensive multidisciplinary scientific journals, publishing more than 3,300 research papers annually.

Sulforophane has also been the subject of numerous studies for its cancer preventative effects; notably from Dr Talalay, a world-renowned expert on phytochemicals and a leading biomedical researcher. Talalay and his team fed broccoli sprout extracts to female rats for five days. They then exposed them and a control group to a carcinogen. The rats that had received the extract developed fewer tumours. Those that did have tumours developed smaller ones that took longer to grow than the control groups did.

Why Broccoli Sprouts Juice?

Broccoli sprouts juice, when extracted properly, is a super source of sulforophane; although I have to admit that it's not a juice that one would normally make at home, since you'd need a large available source of broccoli sprouts in order to extract enough juice to make it worthwhile. That's why I decided to source ready-made unpasteurised broccoli sprouts juice from companies that specialise in its production. There's more information about this under 'Useful Information' at the end of this book, in addition to further information on the subject of juicing.

CHAPTER 4
The Wonderful World of Sprouts

In the preceding chapter, I expounded upon the healing properties of broccoli sprouts. But what do we know about the other exciting sprouting options that are available to us?

Being a vegan who lives solely on fruits and vegetables for twelve months of the year can be quite challenging, especially if you're trying to buy organically-grown produce whenever possible. Of course, this situation will vary according to where you live in the world. For example, there's a big difference between living in the UK compared to the warmer climate of Florida, with the latter providing favourable growing conditions throughout the year.

However, regardless of where you're located on this planet, there is a way of providing yourself with a year-round supply of organically-grown fresh vegetables, albeit in miniature. **Welcome to the wonderful world of sprouts!**

As you'll no doubt now be aware, sprouts are basically tiny plants that grow from the seeds of the 'mother' plant. For example, sunflower seeds from a fully grown sunflower, when planted, grow into young sunflower shoots that can be eaten raw. Another example would be radish sprouts which are grown from the seeds of a radish plant.

Sprouts are a Godsend for Vegans!

One of the reasons that I love eating sprouts is because they're not only one of the most nutritious foods on earth, they're easy to grow and cost effective. Not only this, sprouts can be 10-30 times more nutritious than the best organic vegetables, and unlike commercially-grown vegetables, they're not laced with pesticides, fungicides, herbicides and artificial nitrates.

Another good reason to eat sprouts is because they're easy to digest, since the enzyme-inhibitors will have been removed during the germination process when the seeds are soaked for several hours in water. Also, let's not forget that sprouts contain a rich supply of enzymes that help in the digestive process. Sprouts are also often a good source of protein; for example, sunflower sprouts contain the full range of amino acids needed by the body and unlike animal proteins such as meat, they're easily digested.

Finally, sprouts contain good levels of antioxidants and other natural compounds that help to protect us from the free radical damage that comes about as a result of exposure to pollutants such as radiation, air pollution, stress, damaged fats and processed foods. Free radicals can accelerate the ageing process as a result of cellular damage, and make us more vulnerable to chronic illness.

What About Germination?

Before a seed can develop into a tiny plant, it needs to go through the germination process. This involves soaking the seeds in water for several hours, which releases those naturally occurring enzyme inhibitors that make them difficult for the body to digest.

Once these inhibitors are removed, the seeds begin to come to life as their dormant enzymes become activated. This is when the magic happens because the enzymes convert the inactive nutrients into a nutritional 'elixir' that furnishes the baby plant with everything it needs to begin growing at a rapid rate.

Compared to the majority of plant foods, sprouted seeds are superior in terms of their nutritional value. Firstly, they're often higher in antioxidants, enzymes, amino acids (the building blocks of protein) and other nutrients in comparison with the fully grown plant.

Some of the Most Popular Sprouts

Alfalfa

These are quick-growing and highly nutritious, providing vitamins A, D, E and K.

They are a good addition to salads and sandwiches.

Broccoli

Extremely nutritious and as already mentioned, a fantastic source of the powerful antioxidant sulforophane

Clover

Similar to alfalfa, clover sprouts are a great blood cleanser and a good source of calcium iron, potassium and protein

Fenugreek

Fenugreek sprouts are easy to grow and add a nice aromatic flavour to salads.

They're good for helping to detoxify the colon and are a good source of vitamins A and C plus iron and phosphorous.

Lentils

Lentil sprouts contain about 25% protein and are a good source of vitamin C.

You can sprout any type of lentil, although the Puy variety is probably the best for flavour

They can be sprinkled on soups and used in salads

Mung Bean

Mung bean sprouts are quite well-known to many as they're a familiar ingredient in Chinese cuisine.

They have a nutty flavour and being high in fibre and low in calories, they're great to include in a weight-loss diet. They're also a decent source of vitamin C and iron.

Mustard

Another good one for adding to sandwiches and salads. Similar to radish, they have a spicy kick!

Pea Shoots

Almost all pea varieties will produce pea shoots. Like sunflower, they have a lovely nutty flavour and are high in protein

They're a good source of vitamin C, beta carotene, folate, amino acids and fibre

Pumpkin

You should eat pumpkin seeds sprouts after just a day of sprouting before the shoot appears.

They're a good source of essential fatty acids, B vitamins, vitamin E, phosphorous and zinc. Men who suffer from prostate issues may benefit from eating pumpkin seed sprouts due to their zinc content.

Radish

Radish sprouts have a mild spicy flavour and are great in salads and sandwiches.

They're good source of vitamins A and C.

Sesame

Sesame sprouts are an excellent source of calcium but in a form that is more easily used by the body compared to cow's milk. This is largely due to its content of digestive enzymes and minerals, including magnesium and phosphorous which work in tandem with the calcium.

They're also a good source of B vitamins, E and essential fatty acids

Soybean

A versatile sprout that can be added to cooking but best eaten raw in a salad.

Soybean sprouts are one of the best sources of protein

Sunflower

Sunflower sprouts have a lovely nutty flavour and are excellent when added to salads and as a sandwich ingredient.

They're rich in amino acids, essential fatty acids, some of the B vitamins, vitamin E, iron, calcium, magnesium and potassium.

Quinoa

Quinoa is known as an ancient grain that's often eaten by people who are on a wheat or gluten-free diet. They're also great for vegans since when they're sprouted, they're a good source of protein, B vitamins and vitamin E.

They also have the advantage of being one of the quickest sprouting seeds.

How to Grow Sprouts

There are various types of apparatus that can be used to grow your own sprouts, ranging from a basic glass jar and muslim cloth, to sprouting machines that automatically water the seeds every few hours.

Having tried a range of equipment myself over the years, I think that the good old glass jar method is as good as any for growing good quality sprouts.

All you need is a jar, such as a jam jar that will allow you to place your hand inside. You'll also need a piece of muslim cloth or nylon mesh to cover the top of the jar. This can be held in place with an elastic band. The jar will need to be placed upside down at an angle of 45 degrees. Having said this, you can buy a taylor-made jar that comes with the accessories from several sources, including Amazon.

Method

Soak the seeds in water for the recommended time as shown on the seed packet. This varies according to which seeds you're germinating. When this is done, drain the water and wash the seeds for one minute. After draining thoroughly, place the cloth over the top of the jar and angle upside down at angle of 45 degrees in a pleasant position, preferably at room temperature. Avoid extremes of heat such as near radiators or strong sunlight which may result in the seeds being dried out.

Make sure that you rinse and drain the sprouts once a day for the next 2-5 days until they're ready to eat. This may need to be done twice daily in hot weather.

For more in-depth information on sprouting, I'd recommend that you refer to the excellent book, **Living Foods for Optimum Health: Staying Healthy in an Unhealthy World** by Brian R. Clement with Theresa Foy DiGeronimo; Prima Books. See also under Useful Information at the end of this book.

CHAPTER 5
Fermented Foods:
A Great Option for Vegans

Fermentation is a traditional food preservation technique that can be traced back as far as human history itself, and historians have uncovered signs of it being used in food and beverage preparation as far back as 7000 BC.

In the days before we had mod-cons like fridges and freezers, fermented foods provided humans with food that in some cases proved to be a life-saver. For example, in northern climes when few vegetable crops can be grown during the Winter months, vegetables and fruits that were harvested and fermented during the harvest period were often fermented and stored, thus providing an invaluable source of nutrients when little fresh produce was readily available.Of course, some fermented foods are produced using animal derived products, such as cheese and yoghurt which can be stored for much longer compared to milk, which soon turns sour.

What is Fermentation?

Fermentation takes place as a result of the action of bacteria and sometimes yeasts on a variety of foods. For example, the production of alcohol due to the action of yeasts on grains, goes back to ancient times, becoming so popular that its production may have encouraged humans to begin the farming of grains, such as wheat, barley and rice.

The actual process of fermentation occurs when bacteria (and yeasts) break down and transform a substance into something different, and in so doing, the activity of the microbe's results in distinctive textures and flavours being imparted to the food, as well as enhancing their nutritional profile.

The Benefits of Eating Fermented Foods

Scientists believe that fermented foods are good for our health because they contain live probiotic bacteria with proven benefits for the gut; including normal digestion, increasing the gut's resistance to colonisation of unhealthy bacteria and yeasts, enhanced absorption of nutrients and a healthy immune system.

As a vegan, I find that fermented vegetables can be a great way of adding a bit of variety to my meals, as well as being a good source of nutrients and healthy bacteria. Moreover, fermentation can also neutralise certain plant compounds that sometimes interfere with the absorption of nutrients, such as phytic acid found in wheat and in soya. This can also result in some fermented foods being easier to digest. A classic example being those fermented soya products such as tofu and miso, mentioned in the foregoing.

It's also worth noting that certain bacteria can metabolise natural antioxidants such as polyphenols, increasing their levels. For instance, green tea contains good levels of polyphenols and when the tea is fermented in to a beverage known as kombucha, the polyphenol content is boosted.

Other benefits associated with consuming the bacteria in fermented foods include:

- Production of vitamins, organic acids and short-chain fatty acids
- Creating an unfavourable environment for unhealthy bacteria to grow
- Prevention of digestive upsets
- Restoring the microbiome balance after taking antibiotics
- They can help to maintain the integrity of your gut lining, which helps to prevent foreign substances from passing through the gut wall and getting into your bloodstream, which can trigger an immune response

Bacteria in Fermented Foods

The most common type of microbe found in fermented foods is lactic acid bacteria. Unlike a lot of potentially harmful bacteria, they can live in a salty environment, which is why salt brine is commonly used for fermentation of vegetables such as cabbage and kimchi

Examples of Fermented vegetables

The great thing is that we can ferment virtually any vegetable, including the likes of carrots, asparagus, cabbage and broccoli.

Here's some examples of popular fermented foods and beverages:

Food	Interesting Facts
Vegan 'cheese'	Unlike some of the unhealthy vegan cheeses that I come across in some supermarkets and health food stores; this version is usually made from the likes of cashew nuts that are pre-soaked and whipped into a cream, then fermented using a probiotic culture. You can also get vegan cream cheese made from fermented almond milk.
Cider Vinegar	This is made from fermenting apples and it's best to opt for the raw unpasteurised version containing the 'mother', or original ferment, as this contains the live bacteria that get destroyed in the pasteurised vinegar
Yoghurt	This is probably the most well-known probiotic food that is traditionally made from cow's or goat's milk. However, the good news is that you can purchase a vegan version in the form of almond or soya yoghurt. It's also possible to buy 'live' yoghurts made from oat milk or coconut.

Kefir	Again traditionally a fermented dairy beverage but also available in a dairy-free form. It can be made at home using sugar, water and kefir grains.
Kombucha	This beverage is made from tea, sugar and a culture of bacteria and yeasts. The microorganisms in kombucha transform the sugar into alcohol, acetic acid and vitamins

Top Tip!

Whenever possible choose raw unpasteurised fermented foods, since these products contain the probiotic microbes. Having said this, the pasteurised fermented foods still contain the nutrients that were produced during the fermentation process, so they'll still be good to include in your diet.

If you decide to ferment your own products at home, then that will be an advantage as they'll always be in their raw state, unless you decide to cook them, which is not really advisable

CHAPTER 6
Where Are You on the Health-Disease Spectrum?

I devised this Diet-Disease Spectrum to help those transitioning from a non-vegan diet as a means of determining what changes they need to make in order to promote good health. The spectrum is equally useful for those who are already adhering to a vegan diet.

<< DISEASE .... HEALTH >>

A	B	C	D	E	F	G
Refined carbs such as processed flour, white rice, high sugar/salt, processed meat, dairy and fish substitutes; high saturated fats and trans fats; processed foods (e.g. ready meals; too many starchy vegetables and pulses (e.g. potatoes/chick-peas); vegan sauces containing refined sugars and artificial additives	Refined carbs, high sugar/salt, limited consumption of fermented meat, fish and dairy substitutes; saturated fats and trans fats, processed foods; starchy vegetables; low starchy vegetables (e.g. cabbage, cauliflower, squashes, beets, carrots, etc.). Fresh fruits	Refined carbs, limited wholegrains, nuts/seeds, saturated fats and trans fats, fresh fruits, daily; some high starchy vegetables (e.g. potatoes, most squashes, etc.); fresh fruits	Some refined carbs, some wholegrains, seeds, fruits, healthy fats, approx. 5-6 vegetable portions daily; moderate sugar and salt intake, mostly healthy fats derived from the likes of almond, flaxseed, chia and raw nuts/seeds	Mostly wholegrains, Raw nuts/seeds, fruits, vegetable fats, high raw); fruits, some raw) moderate salt/sugar, pulses, fruits, almond milk, almond yoghurt (naturally sweetened if desired)	Wholegrains, raw nuts/seeds, high vegetable intake (50% raw); fruits, low salt; vegetable intake: 8-10 limited intake of natural low salt; minimal use of natural sugars; superfoods' such as spirulina, Pulses; sprouted seeds (e.g. alfalfa, mung beans, radish)); almond milk, almond yoghurt, coconut kefir, raw cacao	Sprouted nuts/seeds/pulses/grains (e.g. sunflower, snow pea, radish, alfalfa); chlorophyll rich foods comprising largely of leafy greens and green vegetables such as broccoli; high vegetable intake (80-100% raw); very low salt; minimal use of natural sugars; superfoods' such as spirulina, reishi mushrooms; freshly prepared juices, including green juices (e.g. wheatgrass, kale); healthy fats (e.g. omega 3 and 6 from cold pressed flaxseed oil); sea-greens; Food state supplements such as vitamins and mineral derived from plant sources

Here's How it Works:

I devised the health and disease diet spectrum so that you can evaluate how close your current diet is in relation to the holistic view of foods that either, increase your chances of developing disease; or conversely, those foods that enhance your chances of achieving optimum health. As you'll observe, the closer that your diet aligns with the categories towards the right of the table, the better in terms of increasing the chances of achieving a healthy state.

Having said this, the type of diet encompassed within each category may not necessarily exactly match your own; for example, your diet may closely align with category F, whilst not necessarily being an exact match. This doesn't matter too much, as long as you are eating the majority of foods in that category. So, allow for some overlap.

There will also be other factors that may influence health and disease; for example, lifestyle factors such as stress levels, pollution exposure and lack of exercise.

NB. As can be observed from the foregoing spectrum, the diet that encompasses the greatest number of vegetables, predominately in their raw state, is favoured as a means of promoting good health and greatest resistance to diseases such as Alzheimer's, cancer, arthritis and heart conditions. This really stands out when you look at the list of foods in category G.

The evidence for this is backed up by several scientific studies; the most extensive being that of the China Study, which is the most comprehensive study of nutrition ever conducted **(The China Study, Campbell, Colin, T PhD; and Campbell, Thomas, M II).**

I have included a summary of the China Study below:

THE CHINA STUDY - SUMMARY

Summary: *What is The China Study?* It's the largest comprehensive study of human nutrition ever conducted. It was launched via a partnership between Cornell University, Oxford University, and the Chinese Academy of Preventative Medicine. The ground-breaking results from the study recommend a whole food plant-based diet as the best for long-term health. Please note the following observations:

1. **Health Statistics in Western Societies are Frightening.** The increase in adult and child obesity, diabetes, cancer, heart disease and other chronic illness is evidence in itself that that we're doing something very wrong. In addition to increasingly polluted environments, the core of the problem appears to be the very food we eat on a daily basis.

2. **Animal protein promotes the growth of cancer.** The book author T. Colin Campbell, PhD., grew up on a dairy farm, so he regularly enjoyed a wholesome glass of milk. In hindsight, it would appear to be a big mistake. There have been numerous peer-reviewed animal studies that indicate that the casein in milk can actually turn the growth of cancer cells on and off simply by raising and lowering the amount ingested.

3. **The Study Findings are Highly Significant.** After years of controversial lab results on animals, the researchers had to see how they played out in humans. The study they created included 367 variables, 65 counties in China, and 6,500 adults (who completed questionnaires, blood tests, etc.). "When we were done, we had more than 8,000 statistically significant associations between lifestyle, diet, and disease variables."

4. **The Overwhelming Conclusion:** Eat plants for health. People who ate the most animal-based foods suffered from the most chronic disease. People who consumed the greatest amount of plant-based foods were the healthiest.

5. **Carbs are not the enemy.** Highly-processed, refined carbohydrates such as white sugar, white flour and white rice are bad for you. But plant foods are full of healthy carbs bound up by fibre (good for health of the colon) and contain a wide range of nutrients.

6. **Plants are Highly Protective.** It's not just cancer and heart disease that respond to a whole-foods, plant-based diet. It may also help protect you from diabetes, obesity, autoimmune diseases, bone, kidney, eye, and brain diseases.

7. **Plants Are a Good Source of Protein:** A vegan diet if based around a variety of fruits, vegetables, whole grains, nuts and seeds will provide a more than adequate supply of protein. Studies have shown that animal derived proteins encourage the proliferation of cancer cells whilst vegetable proteins don't

8. **Plants are the best source of nutrients.** There are virtually no nutrients in animal-based foods that are not better provided by plants, especially when organically-grown.

CHAPTER 7
The Evidence-Based Healing Properties of Fruits and Vegetables

Having decided to include a chapter in this book on fruits and vegetables and their special properties, I must confess that I didn't know where to begin. After all, there are so many things to mention: healing properties, nutrient content, the range of antioxidants each one contains, and the disease preventing and healing plant compounds (phytochemicals) that are unique to each fruit and vegetable.

After much deliberation, I decided that it wasn't enough to just convey information without including evidence to support the claims. I have, therefore, included a comprehensive list of references at the end of this book under 'Useful Information'.

Apples

"An apple a day keeps the doctor away"

This old saying may seem to be exaggerated folk law, however, modern science continues to validate the medicinal properties of apples. For example, apples have been studied in relation to reducing different forms of cancer, including the following:

- Colorectal cancer (1)
- Breast cancer (2)
- Stomach cancer: It would appear that certain phytochemicals found in apples help to prevent stomach cancer as a result of their inhibition of Helicobacter pylori, an infection that's been linked with stomach ulcers and gastric cancer. Moreover, apple procyanidin has been studied for its ability to directly induce cancer cell death within stomach cells (3)

- It appears that several components of apples bestow beneficial effects. For instance, apple cider vinegar has been found to contain an anti-tumour compound called alpha-glucan which is formed as a result of the fermentation process.

Other beneficial effects from eating apples include the following:

- Diarrhoea: Apple combined with chamomile has been shown to shorten the course of certain types of non-specific diarrhoea.

- Hardening of the arteries (Atherosclerosis): Preclinical research has shown apples contain compounds that prevent the formation of plaque in the arteries (4)

- Overweight: Apples appear to play a part in helping with weight loss

- Radiation Protection: Amazingly, it's been proven that one of the ways that apples help to protect us from cancer is down to their ability to remove radioisotopes that have accumulated in the body. This is a result of fallout from the Chernobyl and Fukishima disasters, in addition to contamination from depleted uranium munitions and other sources. This is due to the pectin content of apples which has been shown to reduce Cesium-137 levels by as much as 60% in exposed children. Apple pectin has also been found to prevent Plutonium-239, one of the deadliest radioisotopes, from being absorbed in the gastrointestinal tract of animals fed on it (5)

Nutritional Value

Apples are a source of:

- Pectin
- Vitamin C
- Potassium
- Calcium

- Copper
- Iron
- Phosphorous
- Magnesium
- Protective phytonutrients such as anthocyanidin

Apricots

Apricots are closely related to peaches and plums and they have long been associated with promoting good health.

This fruit became extremely popular throughout history and this is hardly surprising when we take into consideration their numerous health benefits. This is likely due to them being a good source of unique organic compounds, vitamins and minerals. In addition, the kernel (stone) found in apricots is a wonderful source of apricot oil which has several health benefits.

Other Beneficial Effects
- Strengthens bones: Apricots have almost all the minerals required to build bones; namely, calcium, manganese, magnesium, iron, phosphorous and iron.
- Strengthens the heart and entire cardiovascular system due to its unique nutrient profile that includes vitamin C and Potassium. Vitamin C is known to help protect the heart from free radicals and potassium helps to lower blood pressure
- Apricots are known to have anti-inflammatory properties and are especially good for relieving arthritis
- Anaemia: Since they are an excellent source of iron in a form that the body can easily use to form haemoglobin, apricots are especially good for those suffering from anaemia. In addition, apricots contain copper which aids in iron absorption. What's more, dried apricots are listed as a recommended food for

anaemia on the NHS (National Health Service) Inform website, along with several other foods that are high in iron and other blood-building nutrients.

- Here's the link: https://www.nhsinform.scot/illnesses-and-conditions/nutritional/iron-deficiency-anaemia

NB. When buying dried apricots opt for organically grown fruit when possible. It's also wise to avoid those containing sulphur dioxide, especially if you suffer from asthma as this chemical can trigger asthma attacks in some people.

Nutritional Value

- Apricots are a good source of vitamin A (in the form of beta carotene), C, niacin, K and E
- They also contain essential minerals including potassium, copper, manganese, magnesium and phosphorous
- They are a good source of dietary fibre

Avocados

Avocados come in several varieties with the most popular being the Hass avocado, sometimes referred to as the 'alligator fruit' because of its green knobbly skin. Avocados are a nutrient rich fruit which is high in heart healthy monounsaturated fats, similar to olive oil. They are a good source of vitamin E, which is known as a powerful antioxidant.

Other Beneficial Effects

- Avocados contain lutein and zeaxanthin which exert a protective effect against light waves that can damage your vision. People who eat foods rich in these antioxidants reduce the risk of developing age-related macular degeneration, which is the leading cause of blindness in the older generation

- There is evidence to suggest that avocados help to reduce blood pressure which is a major risk factor for strokes, heart attacks and kidney failure. This is believed to be due to the high level of potassium in the fruit which is higher than in bananas.
- Avocados can lower cholesterol and triglycerides which are blood markers that are linked to an increased risk of heart disease. A number of controlled studies have assessed the effects of eating avocados on some of these risk factors (7). These studies show that avocados raise good cholesterol (HDL) and lower bad cholesterol (LDL)

Nutritional Value

- Avocados are a good source of fibre
- They're high in vitamin and potassium
- They're a good source of protective natural compounds including lutein and zeaxanthin
- They're high in monounsaturated fats, including oleic acid which is also found in olive oil
- They also contain beta carotene, magnesium, vitamin C, K1, B6, folate, niacin and pantothenic acid

Bananas

Bananas are a healthy and delicious fruit and probably the most convenient fruit for snacking. They provide both short-term and long-term energy due to the combination of fruit sugars and resistant starch. Starch takes longer to convert to energy, hence the long-term energy benefits of bananas. Not surprisingly, they are popular with tennis players and other sports participants.

Bananas may also help with weight regulation as a medium sized fruit has about 105 calories.

Other Beneficial Effects

- They're high in potassium which helps to balance electrolyte levels

- In addition to resistant starch, they contain pectin, both of which may help to moderate blood sugar levels after meals

- Bananas are low to medium on the glycaemic index which measures how quickly foods increase blood sugar levels. Having said this, those suffering from Type 2 diabetes are advised not to eat too many ripe bananas due to their sugar content

- They may help to boost your digestion by feeding the healthy bacteria in your gut. This is thought to be due to the presence of resistant starch which acts as food for friendly bacteria

- They may help to protect kidney function due to their high level of potassium

- Bananas are a good source of antioxidants which help to protect us from chronic diseases such as heart disease cancer (8)

Nutritional Value

- They're a good source of potassium, vitamin B6 and vitamin C

- They're an excellent source of easily digestible carbohydrate and fibre

Beetroot

Beets, otherwise known as beetroot, are known to help lower high blood pressure. This is due to beetroot being high in nitrates which your body converts into nitric oxide. Studies have shown that there can be a ten-point drop in systolic blood pressure in volunteers within hours of consuming beetroot juice. This action is due to the fact that nitric oxide has the effect of dilating the blood vessels, thus reducing pressure.

The high nitrate content of beetroot supports the cardiovascular system in other ways too. One study concluded that beetroot juice enhanced the body's tolerance to high intensity exercise (9).

Other Beneficial Effects

- Radiation Exposure: compounds found in beetroots known as betalains, have been shown to exert protective effects against exposure to damaging gamma radiation (10)
- Cancer: beetroot juice has been shown to exhibit anti-cancer properties in prostate cancer cell lines (11)

Nutritional Value

- Beetroot is a good source of folate and B-complex vitamins such as B3 (niacin), B5 (pantothenic acid) and B6 (pyridoxine)
- Fresh roots contain small amounts of vitamin C; however, the top greens are an excellent source of this vitamin in addition to various carotenoids, flavonoids and antioxidants.
- The roots are a rich source of the phytochemical, glycine betaine which has the property of lowering homocysteine levels in the blood. Homocysteine is a toxic metabolite which is associated with a higher risk of developing coronary heart disease.
- Beetroot is a good source of fibre.
- They're a moderate source of potassium

Blueberries

Blueberries are fantastic for our health as they're nutrient-dense, low in calories, high in fibre, rich in vitamin C a great source of antioxidants and protective plant compounds such as anthocyanins, responsible for their deep blue colour and potent health benefits. Compared to many other foods they have one of the highest amounts of antioxidants.

Wild blueberries are even more nutrient dense compared to the commercially grown varieties. If possible, I advise you to opt for organically grown berries whenever available, since most berries are heavily sprayed with pesticides.

As with beetroot, blueberries have been shown to lower blood pressure. This is supported in an interesting article by Dr Mercola. Here's the link:

https://articles.mercola.com/sites/articles/archive/2015/02/02/blueberries-help-lower-blood-pressure.aspx

Other Beneficial Effects

- Skin care: the anthocyanins in blueberries help to prevent DNA damage to the skin from free radicals. Furthermore, their vitamin C content helps in the formation of collagen. Not surprisingly, therefore, regular consumption of blueberries may help to reduce the signs of ageing skin, including reduction of wrinkles and so-called age spots.

- Anti-cancer effects: A report published by the Beckham Research Institute of the City of Hope, California, in the Cancer Research Journal, suggests that blueberries have anti-cancer properties (12)

- Brain Function: It would appear that the combination of vitamins, minerals and phytochemicals in blueberries may protect our brains from free radical damage and as such, there may be positive implications for lowering the risk of suffering from disorders such as Alzheimer's disease and dementia (13)

- Sun Protection: The anthocyanins and other nutrients present in the fruit help to protect us from exposure to UV radiation exposure.

- Weight Loss: Their high fibre content and low calories (around 15g of carbohydrate and 84 calories in one cupful) make them an ideal food for a weight loss programme.

- Urinary Tract Infections: Similar to cranberries which are known for alleviating urinary tract infections, blueberries may also be of benefit since they too contain natural compounds that prevent bacteria from adhering to the walls of the bladder.

- Eye Care: Blueberries may delay age-related ocular problems, including macular degeneration, cataracts and myopia. This is thought to be due to the specific eye-protective antioxidants, lutein, zeaxanthin, along with flavonoids like resveratrol and quercetin.

- Heart Protection: Research has shown that women who ate more than three servings of blueberries per week lowered their risk of having a heart attack by a whopping 32 percent (14)

- Longevity: Plant compounds such as polyphenols and resveratrol found in blueberries have long been associated with increasing longevity and in decreasing the adverse effects linked with advancing age, especially when combined with exercise and good lifestyle habits

Nutritional Value

- A good source of vitamin C, K1 and manganese with smaller amounts of vitamin E, B6 and copper
- They're high in fibre
- They're rich in antioxidants and protective plant compounds, including anthocyanins, quercetin and myricetin

Broccoli

Broccoli is highly revered for its powerful healing benefits. It is an edible green plant in the cabbage family, otherwise known as cruciferous vegetables. Other cruciferous vegetables apart from cabbage include, turnips, Swedes, Brussels sprouts, Bok choy, kale, radishes and cauliflower. They are all high in sulphur, which makes them a good liver supporting food since this organ requires sulphur in one of its detoxification pathways. They also all contain glucosinolates which help the liver to produce enzymes for detoxification.

Broccoli, along with other cruciferous vegetables are a useful source of protein for vegans, especially when eaten raw; for example, chopped and added to a salad, or used as one of the ingredients in a smoothie.

Other Beneficial Effects

- Cancer Prevention: Broccoli is known around the world for its anti-cancer properties. Studies have suggested that this is due to compounds found in broccoli called isothiocyanates which have been shown to affect the liver enzymes, stimulate the immune system and reduce oxidative stress. Moreover, this compound may interfere with the cancer cell's DNA inhibiting its ability to replicate (15)

- As previously mentioned, broccoli also contains a plant compound called sulforaphane which helps to get rid of bacteria called H. Pylori, that can increase the risk of cancer of the stomach. In addition, broccoli provides another natural compound called indole-3-carbinol, which is an anti-carcinogen that is thought to help prevent various types of cancer.

- Antioxidants: Broccoli is a great source of antioxidants that can help the body in various ways, including protecting our cells from the damaging effects of free radicals. Also, the vitamin C found in broccoli helps support the immune system and the flavonoids it contains helps to recycle the vitamin C efficiently. Broccoli is also a good source of the carotenoid's lutein, zeaxanthin and beta carotene

- Bone Health: Broccoli contains high levels of both calcium and vitamin K which are vital for normal bone formation and for prevention of osteoporosis. It also contains other bone-supporting minerals like magnesium, phosphorous and zinc.

- Heart Health: As previously stated, broccoli contains sulforaphane which has been shown to help maintain a healthy heart (16)

- Eye Health: Broccoli contains key nutrients that support eye health, including vitamin C, E, B complex and beta carotene and these may play an important part in helping to prevent macular degeneration and cataracts

Nutritional Value

- Fresh broccoli is a great source of several phytonutrients such as thiocyanates, indoles and sulforaphane
- It contains vitamins K, C, folic acid and potassium
- It's high in fibre
- Brocccoli is quite high in protein at around 2.82 grams per 100 grams.

Cabbage

Cabbage is another member of the cruciferous family of vegetables.

They come in different colours, shapes and sizes; for example, pointed cabbage, red cabbage, white cabbage and savoy cabbage.

Cabbages can be eaten raw in salads (usually grated) and can be used in a variety of ways, including cabbage juice. This sounds a bit gross, but when combined with apple and ginger, it's really quite palatable. In fact, cabbage juice has been shown to help heal ulcers in the gut. This is likely to be due to it containing L-glutamine, S-methylmethionine and glucosinolates which can help protect the stomach and digestive tract by healing the mucous membrane lining.

According to a research paper published in the Western Journal of Medicine, 13 patients with peptic ulcers were treated with fresh cabbage juice and the time to heal the ulcers was a mere 10 days. In stark contrast, patients receiving standard therapy take around 37 days to heal (17)

It's interesting to note that when I was in my teens, I came across a book that mentioned the healing properties of cabbage juice, and it stated that they contain a mystery ingredient known as vitamin U that was known to heal ulcers. Of course, it is likely to be the combination of natural compounds in cabbage that bring about this healing affect.

Other Beneficial Effects

- Anti-Cancer: One of the key cancer- fighting ingredients found in cabbage is sulforaphane and researchers are currently exploring its ability to delay or impede cancer. So far, the results on various types of cancer have been promising (18). There's more on the remarkable healing properties of sulforophane in chapter 3

- Antioxidants: Cabbage contains the key antioxidants, choline, beta-carotene, lutein and quercetin. They all help support the different organ systems in the body; for example, choline can help prevent neural tube defects in pregnant women (19)

- May Promote Heart Health: Red cabbage is rich in anthocyanin, a compound that has been associated with reduced risk of cardiovascular disease (20)

Nutritional Value

- Cabbage is a storehouse of phytochemicals such as thiocyanates, indole3-carbinol, lutein, sulforaphane, isothiocyanates and zeaxanthin

- Fresh cabbage is a good source of vitamin C and vitamins B-1, B-5 and B-6

- Cabbages are also an adequate source of minerals like iron, magnesium, manganese and potassium

- They're an excellent source of **vitamin K** which is important for bone health

Honeydew Melon

Honeydew melon is known for its sweet flesh and aromatic odour. It's very popular around the world and can be eaten by itself or used in desserts, salads, snacks and even in soups.

Honeydew melon is especially valued in countries with a hot climate as it is about 90% water and rich in the electrolytes, potassium, magnesium, calcium and sodium which help to keep us hydrated in hot weather.

Other Beneficial Effects

- Blood Pressure: They may help to lower blood pressure due to their high potassium content

- Healthy Bones: Honeydew melon supplies several nutrients known to help maintain healthy bones, including, folic acid, vitamin K and magnesium. Honeydew also provides small amounts of other bone-supporting nutrients, including calcium, phosphorus and zinc.

- Easily Digested: The fruit sugars in honeydew melons are quickly absorbed by the body and therefore provide a quick boost in energy. This is especially good for athletes prior to a competition or training. Eating honeydew melon after training or an event is also good for recovery

- Immune System: Vitamin C is well known for its role in supporting the immune system and honeydew melon is high in this vitamin. Some evidence suggests that vitamin C may play a crucial role in helping the immune system fight infections such as the common cold (21)

- Diabetes: You might conclude, bearing in mind honeydew's sugar content, that it wouldn't be a good choice for diabetics; however, it appears that it may have a beneficial effect. This is due to the soluble fibre in honeydew, which binds to the sugar molecules and slows down the rate of absorption into the blood stream. Hardly surprising therefore, that it falls into a glycaemic index of 65, despite its sugar content.

Nutritional Value

- It's a good source of vitamin C
- High in soluble fibre
- It's a good source of other vitamins and minerals, including vitamin A, K, folate, B6, potassium, calcium, magnesium, iron and magnesium and zinc (22)
- It contains antioxidants including beta-carotene (which the body converts to vitamin A), phytoene, quercetin and caffeic acid

Carrots

Carrots are a root vegetable which have a good reputation as a health food. They are found in several colours, including yellow, purple, red, white and orange.

They're regarded as a weight-loss- friendly food largely due to them being low on the glycaemic index (G.I) and they're regarded highly for their anti-cancer properties. Carrots have also been linked with improved eye health.

Other Beneficial Effects

- Weight Regulation: Pectin is the main form of soluble fibre in carrots which is good news for diabetics and those trying to shed excess pounds, since soluble fibres slow down digestion of sugar and starch, thus lowering blood sugar levels. They can also feed the friendly bacteria in your digestive system, which in turn not only supports digestion but also your immune system.
- Reduced Cancer Risk: Carrots contain an impressive range of antioxidants and disease-fighting carotenoids, including beta-carotene, lutein, lycopene, polyacetylenes and anthocyanins. Research is on-going regarding their possible effects on cancer cells (23), (24)

- Cholesterol: Carrots would appear to have a cholesterol lowering effect and this may be in part due to their tendency to lower cholesterol absorption from foods (25)

Nutritional Value

- As already mentioned, carrots are a great source of carotenoids, including beta-carotene, which is converted by the body into vitamin A, a vitamin that's important for good eye health

- Carrots also contain biotin (needed for fat and protein metabolism), K1, B6, potassium

- Carotenoids: During the Second World War, fighter pilots suffered from 'night blindness' due to the effects of the powerful searchlights on their eyes. This was remedied when carrots were introduced into their diet. There is also evidence that carotenoids may reduce the risk of age-related macular degeneration (26)

Cauliflower

Like broccoli, cauliflower belongs to the cruciferous family and is highly regarded as an extremely healthy vegetable.

One of the best things about cauliflower is its versatility. It can be used to make cauliflower 'rice', a vegan version of cauliflower 'cheese', roasted in the oven and added to numerous dishes such as casseroles, stir-fries and curries. Personally, I like to use raw cauliflower florets as a salad ingredient.

Cauliflower is associated with several health benefits including reducing the risk of heart disease and cancer. What's more, in common with many other vegetables, cauliflower is anti-inflammatory, which is important because most diseases are thought to be linked with systemic inflammation in the body.

Other Beneficial Effects

- Anti-cancer: In common with other cruciferous vegetables, cauliflower is high in glucosinolates and isothiocyanates, two groups of antioxidants that have demonstrated an ability to slow cancer cell growth (27)

- Weight Regulation: It's a low-calorie vegetable that adds bulk to your meals and is, therefore, a good addition to a weight-control diet. A lot of vegans use pulsed cauliflower as a substitute for rice and legumes when on a low carb diet

- A Source of Choline: Cauliflower is a good source of choline, a vitamin that many people are deficient in. People adhering to a vegan diet should note that cauliflower, along with broccoli, are a good source of choline. Those who don't get enough choline could have a higher risk of heart and liver disease. Moreover, since choline is vital for brain development and for the production of neurotransmitters that are necessary for a healthy nervous system, it may play a role in helping to prevent neurological disorders such as Alzheimer's disease and dementia.

- An impressive source of antioxidants including vitamin C, which is plentiful in cauliflower, although it is depleted when the vegetable is cooked.

- Cauliflower's high sulforophane content may help to reduce high blood pressure and keep arteries in good condition (28)

Nutritional Value

- One of the best sources of vitamin C
- It contains a wide array of vitamins and minerals, including vitamin K, B6, Folate, B5, Potassium, manganese, magnesium and phosphorous
- It is quite high in fibre

- Cauliflower contains a good range of antioxidants that play a significant role in disease prevention. These include isothiocyanates and glucosinolates in addition to carotenoid and flavonoid antioxidants.

Cherries

Cherries are small stone fruits that can be divided into two categories: tart and sweet cherries. They also come in a variety of colours including yellow and deep red.

All varieties of cherries are highly nutritious being a great source of fibre, vitamins, minerals and phytochemicals. They're a good source of vitamin C, which we humans cannot manufacture in the body (unlike like most mammals).

Cherries are especially valued for their plant compounds and anti-inflammatory benefits. This is why they're known to be helpful in inflammatory conditions such as gout and arthritis. People who suffer from these conditions sometimes drink cherry juice to help reduce inflammation. Having said this, benefits may ensue when cherries form a daily part of the diet.

Other Beneficial Effects
- Cherries are especially high in polyphenols, a large group of plant chemicals that help fight cellular damage and reduce inflammation
- Immune System: Their high content of vitamin C helps to support a healthy immune system and protect against free radical damage
- Digestive System: They're a good source of fibre which supports the digestive system by fuelling beneficial gut bacteria

Nutritional Value

- High in vitamin C
- A source of vitamins and minerals including, B vitamins, vitamin K, copper, manganese, magnesium and potassium
- They're a good source of fibre
- They're packed with antioxidants and anti-inflammatory compounds, including polyphenols and beta-carotene

Figs

Figs are a very popular fruit around the world and have been for centuries, which isn't surprising since they are tasty and very nutritious. You can get either green or black figs and out of season they can be purchased in their dried form.

People have used figs for medicinal purposes throughout history. They are purported to help conditions such as constipation, reproductive issues, conditions of the respiratory system and certain skin conditions such as eczema.

Other Beneficial Effects

- Being high in fibre, figs may help to lower cholesterol as well as help control blood sugar levels
- Weight regulation: one large fig has about 47 calories so they're an ideal replacement for unhealthy snacks (in moderation of course).
- Bone Health: Figs are a great plant source of calcium in a form that the body easily utilises; therefore, eating figs on a regular basis may help to reduce the risk of osteoporosis and osteopenia.
- Hair Health: Figs are a popular ingredient in many hair products, including shampoos and conditioners. It's thought that the vitamins and minerals found in figs may help to support the

health of your hair. In fact, one study looked at the role of zinc and copper in relation to hair loss (29). It's thought that zinc may speed up hair follicle recovery. Figs are a good source of zinc

- Protection from Free Radicals: As we know, antioxidants are our main armoury against the free radicals which circulate around the body where they damage our cells resulting in a greater likelihood of disease. According to a 2005 study, dried figs "have superior quality antioxidants" (30)

- Support for the Body's Organ Systems: As already mentioned, figs have been used throughout history to help support the body in a variety of ways, including the endocrine, reproductive, digestive and respiratory systems.

Nutritional Value

- Figs are one of the best plant sources of calcium for vegans.
- They're one of the richest plant sources of vitamins and minerals, including: vitamin A, C, K, B vitamins, potassium, magnesium, zinc, copper, manganese and iron

Flax

Flax seeds have been prized for centuries for their health-promoting properties. In fact, it's known that Charles the Great ordered his subjects to eat flax seeds to keep them healthy. Not surprisingly they acquired the name Linum usitatissimum, meaning "the most useful".

These days flax seeds are highly valued by vegans as a principal source of ALA, a shorter-chain polyunsaturated fatty acid (Omega 3) that the body converts into two different Omega 3 fats; namely, EPA and DHA. These fats have numerous functions in the body; for example, they form a basic component of cell membranes. They provide the starting point for making hormones that regulate blood clotting and the contraction and relaxation of artery walls; they are essential for normal brain function and they help to reduce inflammation in the body.

There is also evidence that regularly consuming flax seeds may lower cancer risk for several cancers including breast, colon, skin and prostate cancer

Other Beneficial Effects

- Flax seeds contain plant compounds known as lignans that act as antioxidants which may help to lower the risk of several types of cancer (31). Flax seeds contain 800 times more lignans than other plant foods
- Breast Cancer: According to some observational studies, those who eat flax seeds have a lower risk of breast cancer, especially postmenopausal women (32)
- Constipation: Flax seeds contain both soluble and insoluble fibre the combination of which ferments in the colon bulking up the stools and helping to counteract constipation
- Lowers Cholesterol: Another benefit associated with regular consumption of flax seeds is their ability to lower cholesterol levels. In one study, people with high cholesterol consumed 3 tablespoons (30 grams) of flax seeds powder daily for three months lowered total cholesterol by 17% and LDL (bad) cholesterol by almost 20% (33)
- Blood Thinner: The Omega 3 rich oil in flax seeds helps to lower the viscosity (thickness) of the blood, thus acting as a natural blood thinner; hence it may help to reduce the risk of blood clots and strokes.

NB. People taking blood thinners such as Warfarin should consult their health practitioner about whether they can also include flax seeds and flax seed oil in their diet

Nutritional Value

- Flax seeds are a good source of lignans
- They are high in soluble and insoluble fibre

- They contain a variety of fats, including saturated, monounsaturated (similar to olive oil), polyunsaturated fats and they are a good source Omega 3 fatty acids
- Flax seeds also contain vitamin B1, B6, folate, calcium, iron, magnesium, phosphorous and potassium

Please also see chapter 10, Key Nutrients for Vegans

Garlic

Garlic is a plant in the Allium (onion) family. It has been used for centuries as a food and medicine. In fact, the Greek physician, Hippocrates, who is sometimes referred to as 'The father of medicine' used to prescribe garlic for a variety of medical conditions.

The latest scientific studies on garlic have indeed confirmed the health benefits that ensue as a result of using garlic either topically, as a food or when taken as a medicine.

Scientists now know that most of garlic's health benefits are caused by sulphur compounds that are formed when a garlic clove is cut into, for example when it is sliced, chopped or chewed. The most famous of these compounds is called **allicin**. This is an unstable compound that is briefly formed in fresh garlic after it's been cut or crushed. Other compounds that may play a role in garlic's health benefits include diallyl disulfide and s-allyl cysteine. The sulphur compounds from garlic are absorbed through the digestive tract after which they circulate around the body where they exert their potent biological effects; for example, helping to destroy harmful bacteria and as a natural blood thinner.

Other Beneficial Effects

- Eating garlic or taking garlic as a supplement is known to support the immune system. A 12-week study concluded that taking a daily garlic supplement reduced the number of colds by a whopping 63% compared to a placebo (34)

- High Blood Pressure: Recent studies have found that garlic supplements help to reduce blood pressure (35). In another study 600-1500 mg of garlic extract was as effective as the drug, Atenolol at reducing hypertension over a period of 24 weeks (36)

- Lowers Cholesterol: It appears that garlic has the ability to lower total cholesterol levels and also LDL (bad) cholesterol by about 10-15% (37)

- Garlic May Offer Protection to the Brain: Antioxidants in garlic may afford protection from brain diseases such as Alzheimer's disease and dementia (38)

- Natural Blood Thinner: Garlic supplements have been shown to naturally thin the blood in a similar manner to aspirin, without the side-effects. They may, therefore, help to reduce the chance of blood clots which can lead to heart attacks and strokes (39)

However, if you're thinking of using them as a substitute for garlic it's important that you first consult your physician. Also, if you have a bleeding disorder, or you're taking anti-coagulant medicine such as Warfarin, it's very important that you consult with your physician before supplementing with garlic.

- Detoxification: Sulphur is known to have a detoxifying effect in the body and this is why garlic is sometimes included as a part of a natural detox programme since it is high in sulphur.

Nutritional Value

- Garlic contains the natural sulphur-based compounds that have several health benefits as already discussed

- It's a good source of vitamin B6, B1 and contains some vitamin C. Garlic also contains the mineral, selenium (known as an anti-cancer mineral). In addition, it has decent amounts of calcium, copper, phosphorous, iron and potassium

Grapes

Grapes come in a variety of colours including black, red, green and even white. Grapes that are eaten as they are or used in a recipe are typically referred to as table grapes, whilst wine grapes are used to make wine. Raisin grapes are usually sun-dried grapes, which as the name suggests, are used to make raisins. All three types belong to the same family, but there are around 60 different species within which there are many varieties.

In addition, you can also get seedless and seeded grapes. In fact, the seeds in grapes are valued because they're a source of grapeseed oil, which is highly valued since it's high in essential fatty acids, especially linoleic acids along with vitamin E.

I first became interested in the health benefits of eating grapes when I came across a fascinating book called The Grape Cure, by a South African lady called Johanna Brandt. She claimed to have cured herself of cancer using grapes as a mono-diet.

The original Brandt Grape Cure Diet was developed by Johanna Brandt in the 1920's. It involves 12 hours of fasting every day, followed by 12 hours where you eat absolutely nothing else except grapes. The rationale behind this protocol is based on the discovery that cancer cells thrive on sugars and when you fast, you're depriving the cancer cells of the sugars they need to proliferate. Subsequently, when you begin consuming grapes after the fast, the cancer cells eagerly consume the sugars from the grapes but at the same time they also take in several natural cancer-killing compounds found in grapes. The type of grape that was preferred were the purple Concord grapes, complete with the skins and seeds.

Other Beneficial Effects

- Longevity: The humble grape may well help us to live a healthier and longer life. This is thought to be due to the phytonutrients that they contain. For example, grapes contain resveratrol, which is a phytonutrient found mostly in the grape skins, grape seeds and the grape flesh. Resveratrol has been shown to increase expression of 3 genes that are related to longevity. In fact, some of the longest-living cultures from around the world, including those who reside in the so-called **blue zones** (40) include grapes in their diets.

- Obesity and Type 2 Diabetes: It seems that polyphenols in grapes may play a role in reducing metabolic syndrome and prevent the development of obesity and type 2 diabetes (41)

- Oxidative Stress: Oxidative stress which can cause damage to our cells and therefore, result in numerous diseases, needs to be kept in check by antioxidants. Grapes are a fantastic source of antioxidants; for example, flavonoids, as a result of their metabolic conversion in the body may produce phenolic acids which have a great capacity to mop up the free radicals that wreak havoc in the body. Other antioxidants in grapes include vitamin C, carotenoids like beta-carotene and phytonutrients like resveratrol.

- Anti-Inflammatory: The body produces inflammation as a protective mechanism against cell injury and invasion of pathogens (e.g. bacteria and viruses). The problem arises if the inflammation persists and becomes chronic inflammation. Such a chronic state can be the underlying cause of diseases such as cancer, cardiovascular diseases, pulmonary diseases, dementia, diabetes and arthritis. The polyphenols in grapes tend to dampen down inflammation. Other natural compounds in grapes, such as proanthocyanidins can impede the pro-inflammatory pathways in the body, thus reducing inflammation. This makes grapes one of the best anti-inflammatory foods around (42)

- Cardiovascular system: The list of benefits to the cardiovascular system from regular consumption of grapes and grape products is very impressive. These include decrease of LDL cholesterol, modulating inflammation and preventing damage to the blood vessel walls. In fact, a recent study that focused upon the effects of a grape extract that was high in resveratrol demonstrated vascular protective effects in patients suffering from coronary artery disease (43)

Nutritional Value

- Grapes are high in fibre.
- They're a good source of vitamin C
- They also supply vitamin K, thiamine, riboflavin, B6, copper, potassium and manganese
- Natural Plant Compounds: Grapes are a fantastic source of phytonutrients including: resveratrol, piceatannol, catechins, epicatechins, procyanidins, proanthocyanidins, viniferones, quercetin, kaempferol, myricetin, caffeic acid, coumaric acid, gallic acid, beta-carotene, lutein and zeaxanthin.

Lemon

Lemons are part of the citrus family, along with the likes of oranges, satsumas, limes and grapefruit.

Citrus fruits are renowned as being a great source of vitamin C and Bioflavonoids. In fact, since the beginning of the 19th century, the Royal Navy decided that they add lemon juice to the sailor's daily ration of grog (watered-down rum). The vitamin C in citrus fruits prevented scurvy.

In a broader sense, research has shown that eating fruits and vegetables rich in vitamin C can reduce your risk of heart disease and stroke (44)

Other Beneficial Effects

- Cholesterol: It appears that citrus fibre may help to lower cholesterol. In one study which involved a group of people taking 24 grams of citrus fibre extract daily for a month, reduced total blood cholesterol levels (45) Plant compounds found in lemons; namely, diosmin and hesperidin have also been found to lower cholesterol
- Lemons are great for detoxifying the liver. Many people drink a lemon and pure water drink first thing in the morning about 20-30minutes prior to having breakfast

- Weight Loss: Research has shown that certain plant compounds in lemons may help reduce weight gain. In fact, in one study, polyphenols extracted from the peel of lemons were fed to mice on a fattening diet and they gained less weight and body fat compared to other mice (46)

- Kidney Stones: Kidney stones are formed from waste products that crystallise and build-up in your kidneys. Citric acid found in citrus fruits may help to prevent kidney stones by increasing the flow of and pH of urine, thus creating a less favourable environment for kidney stone formation (47)

- Protection Against Anaemia: It's been proven that vitamin C helps to enhance the absorption of iron from foods such as spinach and molasses. Therefore, by regularly consuming citrus fruits such as lemons and limes, you will be helping with your absorption of iron and reduce the chances of anaemia

- Cancer Prevention: The plant compounds such as beta-cryptoxanthin and hesperidin found in lemons formed the basis of a study which provided evidence that they may prevent malignant growth developing in the tongues, lungs and colons of rodents (48). More studies are needed to establish whether these benefits are effective against these cancers in humans

Nutritional Value

- Lemons are one of the richest sources in nature of vitamin C

- High in Fibre: The main fibre in lemons is pectin and as we've discovered earlier in this chapter, pectin can lower blood sugar levels by slowing down the digestion of sugar and starch.

- Lemons are a decent source of potassium and B6

- Plant Compounds found in lemons include citric acid, hesperidin, diosmin, eriocitrin and D-limonene. These phytochemicals have been shown to have powerful healing effects on cancer, inflammation and cardiovascular problems

Mango

Sometimes called the 'king of fruits', mango is classed as a drupe, or stone fruit. There are hundreds of types of mango, varying in size, shape and flavour. This fruit is highly valued for its succulent flavour and for its nutritional benefits. For example, mango is packed with antioxidants such as polyphenols. In fact, it has over a dozen types, including catechins, anthocyanins, quercetin, kaempferol, mangiferin, benzoic acid and rhamnetin. As stated earlier in this chapter, antioxidants are our body's protectors as they help to neutralise the highly reactive free radicals that damage our cells.

One polyphenol in particular, mangiferin, has been the centre of a lot of attention and it's regarded as a 'super antioxidant' since it's especially powerful (48) and believed to offer protection against some cancers, diabetes and several other diseases

Other Beneficial Effects

- Boosts the Immune System: Mango is a powerful source of immune boosting nutrients, including vitamin C and beta-carotene. The fruit also contains folate, vitamin E, K and some B vitamins which also support the immune system

- Supports Heart Health: Mango contains certain nutrients that may support a healthy heart, in particular, magnesium and potassium, which help to maintain a healthy pulse and lower blood pressure. Moreover, the antioxidant mangiferin found in mango, may protect heart cells from free radical damage, apoptosis (controlled cell death) and inflammation (49). In addition, it may also help to lower blood cholesterol and triglycerides

Nutritional Value

- Mango is a good source of minerals, including potassium, copper, manganese and magnesium. It also contains smaller amounts of selenium, calcium, iron and phosphorous

- It's a valuable source of vitamins including K, C, folate, niacin, riboflavin, thiamine, B5, B6, A and E.
- As already mentioned, mango is a wonderful source of disease-fighting and health protecting antioxidants

Mushrooms

Mushrooms have been used for food and medicine for hundreds of years. They're particularly valued by the Chinese who have studied their medicinal effects more than any other country. In fact, mushrooms are a key herbal product in traditional Chinese medicine (TCM).

It's known that mushrooms contain powerful phytochemicals that help support immune function, reduce inflammation, protect the liver, have an anti-viral effect and may help to maintain brain health.

According to world-renowned mycologist, Paul Stamets, who has written 6 books on the subject; of the 140,000 species of mushroom-forming fungi, remarkably, science is only familiar with 10%.

Although mushrooms are often highly valued by consumers around the world, many people, vegans included, tend to stick to the ones that they're familiar with; for example, button mushrooms. However, I believe that this is now changing with a wider variety becoming more commonplace in supermarkets. Varieties such as shitake, maitake and cordyceps have become more accepted by consumers in the likes of the USA, European countries and the UK.

According to well respected natural health expert, Dr Mercola, it's important to choose organically grown mushrooms because they tend to absorb whatever they're grown in, whether good or bad. In this regard, mushrooms are known to concentrate toxins such as heavy metals (for example mercury and lead) in addition to toxins that have polluted the air and water.

IMPORTANT!

If attempting to collect wild mushrooms be sure to seek expert advice since some fungi can be poisonous.

Some Examples of Medicinal Mushrooms and Their Health Benefits

- Shitake: A richly flavoured mushroom that helps to boost the immune system (50). They have also been shown to have anti-cancer properties (51) and anti-inflammatory properties

- Maitake: Another mushroom with an intense flavour. They're known as an adaptogen. Adaptogens help the body to resist stresses such as exposure to toxins and anything that challenges the immune system. Maitake extracts have been studied for their potential benefits in relation to a wide range of conditions, including joint inflammation, septic shock and asthma (52)

- Lions Mane: These are large, white mushrooms that resemble a lion's mane. They're valued for their medicinal and culinary uses in Asian countries like China, India and Japan. For vegans who are missing the flavour of seafood, they have a flavour described as 'seafood-like' and comparable to crab or lobster (53)

Lion's mane mushrooms contain natural compounds that have beneficial effects on the brain, heart and digestive system.

For example, studies have discovered that lion's mane mushrooms contain 2 special natural compounds that stimulate the growth of brain cells; namely, hericenones and erinacines (54)

Nutritional Value

Different mushrooms have different nutritional profiles; however, generally they're a good source of vitamins and minerals, including B vitamins: thiamine, B2, B6 and folate. Most mushrooms contain iodine, iron, copper, magnesium, manganese, selenium, phosphorous, vanadium and zinc. They're also, a good source of fibre, vitamin C and D.

Onions

Onions belong to the Allium genus along with garlic, scallions, chives and leeks. Onions are valued for their medicinal properties as well as their versatility in cooking.

Basically, there are three types of onions: red, yellow and white. They can be eaten raw or cooked, although red onions are usually the preferred choice as a raw food addition to salads, sandwiches, etc. This is because of their milder and less pungent taste.

Onions are a great source of health-promoting phytochemicals, including quercetin, which is an anti-inflammatory compound. It would appear that red onions have the highest number of antioxidants, including quercetin and anthocyanins which provide benefits in protecting against a wide range of diseases.

Other Beneficial Effects

- Like garlic, onions are known to have anti-microbial properties
- The sulphur compounds found in onions help the liver with detoxification
- Onions have been shown to naturally thin the blood and therefore afford some protection against the formation of blood clots which can be life-threatening

Nutritional Value

- Onions are a good source of vitamin C, a nutrient involved in regulating collagen production, supporting the immune system, tissue repair and iron absorption
- Fibre: Onions are rich in soluble fibres called fructans which are sometimes referred to as prebiotic fibres because they feed beneficial bacteria in the gut
- Onions are a rich source of the B vitamins Folate and B6 in addition to being a good source of potassium

- Phytochemicals: Onions are a fantastic source of natural plant compounds including 25 different varieties of flavonoid. Red onions are a particularly good source of special plant pigments called anthocyanins which give red onions their colour.

Oranges

On a trip to Spain many years ago, I remember seeing my first orange tree and was in awe of how beautiful it looked. Each orange seemed to embody the very sunshine that helped its creation; in fact, oranges are sometimes called the 'sunshine fruit'.

Of course, like lemons and limes, oranges are part of the citrus family and in common with the other citrus fruits, they contain a high level of vitamin C along with bioflavonoids that are particularly concentrated in the pith just under the skin.

Oranges are also a decent source of other nutrients as well as natural compounds such as hesperidin, a citrus flavonoid that is one of the main antioxidants found in the fruit. Their rich colour is due to their high content of carotenoids; for example, beta-cryptoxanthin, which your body converts into vitamin A. This is especially important for vegans as non-vegans can derive already converted vitamin A from eating certain animal products such as beef liver.

Orange Juice

Orange juice is one of the world's most popular fruit juices; however, these days it does get something of a bad press due to its high fructose content. My view is that there are health benefits associated with drinking orange juice, providing that you dilute it with pure water (preferably on a 50:50 basis) and you choose organically grown oranges to make your own juice, or opt for fresh unpasteurised juice

Other Beneficial Effects

- Heart Health: Flavonoids in oranges, especially hesperidin, may exert protective effects against heart disease (55). Moreover, some studies have shown that by drinking orange juice over a period of 4 weeks has a blood-thinning effect and may significantly reduce blood pressure (56)

- Kidney stones: These are caused by a build-up of mineral deposits in the kidneys and it appears that orange juice may help to prevent this from happening since it helps to make the urine more alkaline and studies have indicated that a more alkaline urinary pH the less chance of kidney stone formation (57)

- Anti-inflammatory: Inflammation is the body's natural response to infection, injuries, etc. However, if the inflammatory process is sustained and not 'switched off' it is thought to be the cause of many illnesses; including, heart disease, some cancers and arthritis. One study found that orange juice possesses anti-inflammatory properties as a result of reducing anti-inflammatory markers in the body that are associated with chronic disease (58)

Nutritional Value

- In addition to its high vitamin C content, oranges are also a rich source of folate which is needed for synthesis of DNA and for normal foetal development

- Oranges are an excellent source of potassium and as already stated, this is really important for regulating blood pressure and prevention of bone loss.

- Antioxidants: Oranges are a great source of several different antioxidants, including flavonoids and carotenoids which are thought to be essential for disease prevention

Pineapple

Pineapple has to be one of my favourite tropical fruits. Not only is it delicious, it really packs a punch when it comes to its nutritional value and health benefits. These include, possible support for arthritis sufferer (largely due to its anti-inflammatory effects) and help with weight loss. Pineapples have even been used to help eradicate parasites that inhabit the digestive system.

Other Health Benefits

- Digestion: pineapples help to support the digestive process due to the fact that they contain a digestive enzyme called bromelain which helps to break down protein molecules into amino acids, which are the building blocks that the body uses to repair tissue, build hormones and neurotransmitters in the brain and a myriad of other functions in the body. Moreover, they can be especially helpful for people with pancreatic insufficiency, which is when the pancreas isn't producing enough digestive enzymes (59)

- Boosts the Immune System: Pineapples have been used as a medicinal fruit for hundreds of years. They contain a wide range of nutrients including vitamins, minerals, enzymes and antioxidants that may work together to support immunity and suppress inflammation. One study showed that children who ate the most pineapple had a significantly lowered risk of succumbing to both viral and bacterial infections. It was also discovered that the children who ate the most pineapple had almost four times more white blood cells (granulocytes) which fight disease (60)

- Recovery after Surgery and Strenuous Exercise: When we think about it both surgery and strenuous exercise result in damage to tissues which the body sets out to repair. Eating pineapples may accelerate this process, largely as a result of the anti-inflammatory properties of bromelain. In fact, a number of studies have shown that bromelain may reduce the bruising, swelling and pain that occurs after surgery due to the inflammation generated at the site of injury (61)

- Cancer: Consuming pineapple on a regular basis may help to reduce cancer risk. This may be due to the fact that cancer is commonly linked with chronic inflammation and oxidative stress and pineapples contain compounds that help to these two factors. This is borne out by several studies, including two test-tube studies that showed that showed that bromelain suppressed the development of breast cancer cells and stimulated cell death which is known as apoptosis (62)

Nutritional Value

- Pineapples are low in calories which is good for supporting a weight-loss Programme

- They're a great source of vitamin C which supports the immune system as well as acting as a powerful antioxidant

- Pineapples are a really good source of vitamins and minerals, including B6, Thiamine, folate, niacin, Pantothenic acid, riboflavin, magnesium, iron, potassium, copper and manganese. They also contain trace amounts of vitamins A and K

- Antioxidants: Pineapples are a good source of disease-fighting antioxidants, including flavonoids and phenolic acids, Furthermore, some of the antioxidants found in pineapple are bound, which means that they can survive unfavourable conditions in the body resulting in them having longer lasting effects

Prunes

Prunes, or dried plums are extremely nutritious, offering a number of health benefits, including helping with bowel movements when constipation is a problem, and supplying the nutrients that help with osteoporosis, or weakening of the bones.

Prunes and plums contain an impressive range of vitamins and minerals in addition to antioxidants and fibre.

Other Health Benefits

- Constipation: I've often wondered why prunes are so effective in helping overcome constipation. What is it about prunes that makes them different from a lot of other fruits in this respect? Well, we know they're high in fibre with one prune providing around 1 gram of fibre. This adds bulk to your stool and that speeds up the rate that waste moves through your digestive tract. However, I was surprised to discover that prunes contain sorbitol, which is a sugar alcohol that acts as a natural laxative. In fact, it is so effective that eating too many prunes may result in diarrhoea.

- Anti-inflammatory Effects: Prunes are rich in antioxidants and in particular, natural plant compounds known as polyphenols, which exert powerful anti-inflammatory effects, including that of improving bone health and helping to reduce the risk of diabetes and heart disease (63)

- Heart Health: It appears that consuming plums and prunes on a regular basis may help to protect our cardiovascular system. They have been studied for their potential to reduce high blood pressure and cholesterol levels; both factors in heart disease. One study in particular involved subjects who drank prune juice and ate 3-6 prunes each morning for eight weeks. They were compared to a group that drank a glass of water on an empty stomach. It was observed that those who consumed the fruit juice and ate the prunes on a daily basis had lower total cholesterol as well as the so- called "bad" LDL cholesterol in addition to lower blood pressure levels (64)

Nutritional Value

- Prunes contain an impressive range of vitamins and minerals, including vitamin A, C, K, B2, B3, B6, potassium, copper, manganese, magnesium and phosphorus.

- They're high in soluble fibre which supports normal bowel function. They also contain sorbitol which is a natural laxative

- They're a rich source of antioxidants, especially polyphenols, which may support bone health, diabetes, reduce inflammation and help to reduce the risk of heart disease (65)

Strawberries

Strawberries are visually inviting with their beautiful bright red colour, unique aromatic odour and wonderful taste. They're also very versatile and can be eaten on their own, added to breakfast cereals, added to smoothies and used as a flavouring; for example, when making a healthy home-made vegan ice-cream. In terms of our health, strong scientific evidence exists that daily consumption of berries such as blackberries, blueberries and strawberries provide us with several health benefits, such as beneficial effects on the brain, including possible prevention of age-related memory loss and other changes.

Of course, all of these berries possess their own unique nutritional properties, and strawberries are no exception. Their high level of vitamin C and other antioxidants may help to explain why they bestow so many health benefits, such as improving skin health and helping with weight regulation, the latter being due to their content of both soluble and insoluble fibre.

Other Health Benefits

- Reduces Inflammation: It's been shown that strawberries reduce blood levels of C-reactive protein, which is a substance that is produced by the liver that increases inflammation in the body. This was shown in a study conducted by prestigious Harvard School of Public Health which revealed that women who ate more than 16 strawberries in a week were 14% less likely to have elevated levels of C-reactive protein (66)

- Weight Loss: Strawberries boost the fat-burning hormones adiponectin and leptin. In addition, they help reduce appetite and decrease blood sugar, all of which helps to reduce body weight and fat.

- Osteoarthritis: It's been shown that polyphenols and other bioactive compounds found in berries help to ameliorate pain and inflammation in osteoarthritis, the most common form of the disease (67)
- Birth Defects: Strawberries contain folic acid which has been shown to help prevent birth defects. Therefore, consuming them during pregnancy may help to ensure optimal health for mother and baby
- Cardiovascular Health: Several human studies have shown that strawberries in common with other berries, help to improve cardiovascular health. Regular consumption was found to lower LDL ('bad' cholesterol) and to help prevent deposition of cholesterol in the arteries as well as helping to reduce high blood pressure (68)

Nutritional Value

- Strawberries contain lots of vitamin C and are actually a better source of this nutrient than oranges
- Apart from vitamin C, key nutrients found in strawberries include, folate, manganese, potassium and to a lesser extent, iron, copper, magnesium, phosphorus and vitamins B6, K and E
- Antioxidants and Other Plant Compounds: Strawberries are loaded with lots of beneficial antioxidants and other plant compounds, including Ellagic acid, pelargonidin (this gives strawberries their bright red colour) and procyanidins, all of which are believed to provide us with a range of health benefits. In addition, strawberries contain more than 25 different anthocyanidins, with pelargonidin being the most abundant. Overall, this makes the humble strawberry one of the healthiest berries to include in your diet.

Tomatoes

Many people mistakenly consider tomato to be a vegetable but technically speaking it's a fruit.

Of course, tomatoes are widely use in cuisines around the world, and no wonder, as it's incredibly versatile. For instance, they can be used to improve the flavour of food, eaten on their own as part of a salad, used to make sauces as is common in Mediterranean countries, and used as a topping on pizzas. Moreover, tomatoes are easy to cultivate and this is one of the reasons why they're so widely used around the world.

Tomatoes are part of the nightshade family and it would appear that they may aggravate some people who suffer from inflammatory conditions, such as arthritis and gout. This is thought to be due to the presence of specific toxic compounds that are present in nightshades such as tomatoes, peppers, aubergine and potatoes. Although there appears to be no consistent evidence that tomatoes make arthritic conditions worse; it is worth noting that eating lots of tomatoes can cause an increase in uric acid levels in the body which are associated with causing gout, a type of arthritis. As for tomatoes worsening the symptoms in other types of arthritis; the jury is still out on that one. However, I would caution people who suffer from inflammatory conditions such as arthritis, not to eat them in excess.

Of course, on a positive note, tomatoes are a highly nutritious fruit and it's health benefits include helping to manage diabetes, urinary tract infections, improving digestion, improving fluid balance and protection of the kidneys.

Other benefits

- Cardiovascular Health: Studies have shown that the antioxidants, beta carotene and lycopene, which are both abundant in tomatoes, help to protect us from heart disease (69)
- Cancer Prevention: Observational studies have noted links between consumption of tomato products with fewer incidences

of prostate, lung and stomach cancers (70). A study in women showed that high concentrations of carotenoids, such as those found in tomatoes may protect against breast cancer (71)

- Skin Health: Plant compounds found in tomatoes have been shown to promote skin health particularly in relation to their lycopene content. It also seems that tomatoes exert a protective effect against sun burn and may reduce the signs of skin ageing and reduce the occurrence of skin cancer (72). According to one study, people who ingested 1.3 ounces of tomato paste, providing 16 mg of lycopene with olive oil daily for 10 weeks experienced 40% less sunburn.

Watermelon

Watermelon is delicious and the perfect fruit to eat during hot weather, since It's so refreshing and only contains around 46 calories per cup. This makes it a good addition to any calorie restricted diet.

Of course, we know that drinking plenty of pure water is really important to keep our bodies hydrated; nevertheless, sometimes people forget that eating foods that have a high-water content also help to ensure that we don't become dehydrated. Interestingly, watermelon is 92% water.

Undoubtedly, watermelon is also good for our health as it contains a good supply of vitamin C and beta carotene, which is, if you remember, converted to vitamin A by the body. Vitamin A helps to keep our lungs healthy, helps to support eye health as well as being crucial for many other bodily functions

Other Health Benefits

- Weight Regulation: As already mentioned, watermelon is low in calories and has a high-water content, which, along with its high fibre content, helps to keep us full for longer.
- Good for Athletes: This fruit is a good pre-workout and post workout Fruit; again, this is due to its high-water content which

helps to prevent dehydration. When athletes become dehydrated their performance is adversely affected

- Antioxidants: Watermelon contains a wide range of antioxidants, including vitamin C, beta carotene and lycopene

- Anti-inflammatory: Watermelon also contains a plant compound called Cucurbitacin E which has anti-inflammatory and antioxidant effects

- Blood Pressure: Watermelon contains citrulline, an amino acid that may increase nitric oxide levels. Nitric oxide causes the blood vessels to expand, which in turn lowers blood pressure (73).

- Eye-Health: Watermelon's lycopene content may support eye health as it's been found that this plant compound has been found in several parts of the eye where it helps to lower inflammation and protect against oxidative damage. It may also help to prevent age-related macular degeneration (AMD); a common eye problem that can cause blindness in older adults (74)

- Heart Health: Several nutrients in watermelon have been shown to support heart health, including lycopene, which, as we've already observed, may help to reduce high blood pressure. Other nutrients found in watermelon that are good for your heart are vitamins A, B6, C, magnesium and potassium (75)

Nutritional Value

- Watermelon is a good source of vitamin C

- It's a great source of beneficial plant compounds as mentioned in the foregoing

- Compared to many other fruits, watermelon is one of the lowest in calories (around 46 calories per cup), which is even lower than recognised low sugar fruits such as berries

- In addition to its vitamin C content, watermelon is a good source of vitamins B1, B5 and B6 in addition to the minerals, Potassium and magnesium

CHAPTER 8
My 7 Day Vegan Alkaline Diet

The following 7 day alkaline-forming diet for vegans is great for implementing a periodic detox. Moreover, if adhered to for longer, it may help the body overcome some health conditions, such as joint soreness, headaches/migraines, low mood, low energy and numerous other complaints.

Caution: Before embarking upon a detoxification diet of any duration, it's wise to seek the advice of a qualified health physician who will support you through any detoxification symptoms. This is important, since people vary with regard to their toxicity levels, and those with high levels may experience uncomfortable symptoms such as nausea, joint pains and headaches.

Day 1

Breakfast

Quinoa Porridge

Serves 1-2
- 150g quinoa flakes
- 60ml freshly pressed apple or pear juice
- ¼ tsp mixed sweet spice – if desired
- 180ml water

1. Place the quinoa, water and apple juice in a medium-sized saucepan. Bring the mixture to the boil then simmer for around 8 minutes.

2. Turn off the heat, stir-in the spice if desired, and allow to cool before serving

Lunch

1 large salad (see Dave's Super Salads for salad ideas)

Evening Meal

MAIN MEALS

Mediterranean Rice

Serves 1-2

- 1 tbsp of extra virgin olive oil or coconut oil
- 1 medium sized onion (chopped)
- 1 garlic glove (crushed)
- 50g chopped red or green pepper
- ½ tsp of mixed dried herbs
- 300ml water
- 60g of long-grain wholegrain organic rice or similar
- 125g of tomatoes (chopped and peeled) or use organic canned version

1. Gently heat the olive oil in a frying pan and sauté the onion, garlic, mixed herbs and pepper until tender.
2. Add the water, pepper, tomatoes and rice. Cover and simmer for around 25 minutes.
3. Serve when the rice is done.

Or

Mediterranean Roasted Vegetables

Serves 1-2

- 1 orange or red pepper (cut into pieces)
- I yellow pepper (cut into pieces)
- 2 medium sized courgettes/zucchini (Sliced)
- 1 red onions (peeled and cut into quarters)
- 1 Fennel bulb (sliced) - optional
- 2 garlic cloves
- 3 tomatoes (cut into halves)
- 1 aubergine
- Fresh rosemary or dried mixed herbs
- 1 tbsp extra virgin olive oil or coconut oil
- Freshly ground, black pepper.

1. Preheat the oven to 225°C/425°F/Gas mark 6
2. Layer the onions, peppers, tomatoes, courgettes, fennel and aubergine in an oven-proof roasting dish which has been lightly oiled
3. Place the garlic cloves in amongst the vegetables and lightly coat them with olive oil.
4. Place some sprigs of rosemary amongst the vegetables or sprinkle dried herbs
5. Sprinkle with the black pepper.
6. Roast for around 25 minutes, remembering to turn the vegetables at the half-way stage.
7. Makes a great accompaniment to lightly seasoned cooked quinoa.

Breakfast

Fresh Fruit Salad and Coconut Cream or Unsweetened Almond Yoghurt

This is a light and refreshing breakfast with the tangy flavours of the fruit contrasting nicely with the coconut cream or almond yoghurt.

Serves 1

- 1 breakfast bowl of your favourite fresh fruit, sliced
- 1 small carton of almond yoghurt or a little coconut cream
- 1 tbsp of finely chopped nuts
- Layer the sliced fresh fruit into the bowl

1. Pour the cream or yoghurt over the fruit
2. Sprinkle with the chopped nuts and serve

Lunch

Dave's Super Salad (or choose from Salad recipes at the end of this plan)

Evening Meal

Vegetable Stew

Serves 1-2

- ½ red or green pepper (deseeded and sliced)
- ¼ medium sized butternut squash; or sweet potato (peeled and cut into small chunks)

- 1 courgette (sliced)
- ¼ cup of garden peas
- 1 onion (peeled and chopped)
- 1 small can of organic tomatoes
- Chilli powder
- ½ cup of cabbage (chopped)
- 1 clove of garlic (peeled and finely chopped)
- 250 ml of gluten-free vegetable stock
- Pinch of sea-salt
- Ground black pepper
- 1 tbsp extra virgin olive oil

1. Gently heat the oil in a large saucepan
2. Add the onion and garlic and fry for around 3 minutes.
3. Except for the canned tomatoes and chick peas, add the vegetables and fry for a further 10-12 minutes.
4. Add the stock, chilli powder (optional)

Day 3

Breakfast

Porridge made with soaked seeds and Organic Apricots

Prepare the porridge as you would normally and add a little unsweetened almond milk or pure water. Add the soaked seeds and apricots before serving

Lunch

Dave's Super Salad or choose from salad selection at the end of this plan

Evening Meal

Vegetable Stir-Fry

Serves 1-2

- 1 onion (peeled and chopped)
- 2 carrots (peeled and sliced)
- 1 glove of garlic (peeled and sliced)
- 1 red pepper (deseeded and sliced)
- 1 courgettes/zucchini (sliced)
- 1/4 cauliflower (cut into chunks)
- 250g of beansprouts
- 1 sweet potato (peeled and chopped)
- 1 can of chopped organic tomatoes
- 2 tbsp of extra virgin olive oil
- 1 tbsp of gluten-free tamari sauce
- Pinch of sea-salt
- Pepper

1. Heat the oil in the wok and when it is hot, add the onion and garlic. Fry for around 3 minutes.
2. Add the tamari sauce, seasoning and all the vegetables except the beansprouts
3. Fry the vegetables for around 6-8 minutes before adding the beansprouts. Cook for a further 2 minutes.
4. Serve with a little whole grain organic rice or quinoa, if desired

Day 4

Breakfast

Spicy Dried Fruit and Almond or Coconut Cream Yoghurt Delight

Serves 1-2

- 3 tbsp of mixed vine fruit (soaked the night before)
- 285ml plain almond yoghurt or coconut cream
- 1 tsp of sweet mixed spice powder

1. Place an equal amount of the soaked dried fruit into two breakfast bowls and layer with the yoghurt or coconut cream
2. Sprinkle with the sweet spice powder and serve

Lunch

Dave's Super Salad or choose from the salad options at the end of this plan

Evening Meal

Carrot, Swede and Potato Mash

Serves 1-2

- 1/2 medium sized Swede (peeled and diced)
- 2 carrots (peeled and sliced)
- 1 sweet potato (peeled and cut into quarters)
- 1 tbsp of olive oil
- 1 small pot of almond yoghurt

- 1/4 tsp of sea-salt
- Freshly ground black pepper

1. Place the sweet potato, diced Swede and sliced carrots in a pan of water. Bring to the boil and simmer for 10 minutes until the vegetables are thoroughly cooked
2. Add the seasoning and yoghurt and mash until smooth and creamy
3. Serve with any extra vegetables as desired; example, asparagus or green beans. For protein add some naturally flavoured tofu

Day 5

Breakfast

Home-Made Muesli

Mix the following flaked cereals:
- 2 cups of rolled oats
- 2 cups of buckwheat flakes
- 2 cups of quinoa flakes
- 1 cup of rice flakes
- Now add the following seeds:
- 2 tbsp of pumpkin seeds
- 2 tbsp of sesame seeds
- 3 tbsp of shelled hemp seeds

1. Transfer the ingredients to an air-tight container. Serve with almond yoghurt, almond milk or rice milk and sweeten with a little raw honey, coconut sugar or stevia if desired.

Lunch

Dave's Super Salad or choose from the salad list at the end of this plan

Evening Meal

Mixed Vegetable Soup

Serves 1-2

- 2 courgettes/zucchini (sliced)
- 1 large onions (peeled and chopped)
- 2 carrots (peeled and sliced)
- 2 cups of shredded white cabbage
- 2 cups of broccoli florets
- 1 clove of garlic (peeled and sliced)
- ½ cup of Swede of Celeriac (peeled and chopped)
- 5 tsp of organic tomato paste (no citric acid)
- 2 tsp of curry powder or chilli powder (Madras curry powder from the Sainsbury's range is good and it has no salt added
- 1 tbsp of olive oil or coconut oil
- ¼ tsp of sea-salt
- 2 tablespoonsful of organic cider vinegar (with the Mother is best)

1. Place all of the vegetables in a saucepan of water and lightly cook until soft
2. Pour the vegetables and water into a liquidiser and add the cider vinegar and olive or coconut oil. Add some curry powder or chili powder and sea salt and blend until smooth
3. Serve with a slice of rice bread or corn bread spread with a little non-hydrogenated margarine

Breakfast

Rice Pudding

Serves 1-2

- 150g of whole grain organic rice
- 250ml of almond or rice milk (unsweetened)
- Juice of 1 lemon
- 1/4 tsp of cinnamon powder
- 1/2 tsp of stevia or raw honey

1. Place the rice and the other ingredients in a large saucepan. Bring to the boil, lower the heat and simmer for around 15
2. Serve hot, or chill in the refrigerator and eat as a cold pudding

Lunch

Dave's Super Salad or choose one from the salad recipe list

Evening Meal

Ratatouille

Serves 1-2

- 2 courgettes (diced)
- 1 aubergines/eggplants (diced)
- 1 green peppers (deseeded and sliced) - optional
- 1 onion (peeled and chopped)
- 1 garlic clove (peeled and sliced)

- 1 large can of chopped organic tomatoes (no citric acid)
- 2 tbsp of tomato paste (no citric acid)
- ½ tsp of stevia
- 1 tbsp of extra virgin olive oil
- 1 tbsp of mixed fresh or dried herbs
- ½ tsp of sea-salt
- Freshly ground black pepper

1. Place the diced courgettes and aubergines in a colander, sprinkle with the salt, cover, and leave for 15 minutes. Rinse and drain
2. Gently fry the onions and garlic in a large saucepan for 3-4 minutes. Add the green peppers and the drained courgettes and aubergine. Mix well, then fry for 3-4 minutes
3. Add the chopped tomatoes and tomato paste, cover, then gently cook for a further 20 minutes
4. Add the stevia and seasoning and mix well before serving
5. A great combination with an organic baked potato

Alternatively, for quickness, lightly steam or boil a combination of your favourite vegetables and serve with an organic baked potato and some Whole Earth baked beans

Day 7

Breakfast

1 portion of Grain-Free Granola (e.g. from the Paleo Company) with a little almond or rice milk

Dave's Super Salads or choose from the salad list

Evening Meal

Nutty Sweet Potato Burgers

Serves 2

- 225g of potatoes (peeled)
- 1 medium sized red onion (peeled and sliced)
- 115g of mushrooms (washed and sliced)
- 2 tbsp of dairy-free margarine
- 2 tbsp of extra virgin olive oil or coconut oil
- 115g of chopped nuts (of your choice)
- 1 tbsp of parsley
- Pinch of sea salt
- Freshly ground black pepper

1. Boil the peeled potatoes
2. Whilst the potatoes are cooking sauté the onion and mushrooms in the oil
3. When cooked, mash the potatoes with the margarine and season
4. Stir in the cooked onion, mushrooms and the chopped nuts
5. Form into burger shapes
6. Brush lightly with oil and grill
7. Serve with your favourite cooked vegetables or salad

Daily Salad Ideas

I formulated the following mixed salad which can act as a core daily component when planning a healthy vegan diet. This is followed by some specific ideas for other salads at the end of the chapter.

Dave's Super Salad

The good thing about this salad is that it's basic and doesn't need any fancy Preparation.

All you have to do is shred or chop your favourite raw vegetables and place them in a large bowl. If you prepare a large bowl of this salad you can store it in the fridge for 24 hours and it will supply you with several smaller salads during that period.

Here are some ideas for ingredients:

Raw cauliflower	courgettes/zucchini
Tomatoes	spring onions
Red cabbage	white cabbage
Carrot (1 medium)	red and white onions
Sprouted seeds*	Sprouted pulses
Lettuce (all kinds)	Watercress
Seaweeds from Iceland/Norway	
Celeriac	Kohl rabi
Celery	chicory
Mixed green leaves	baby spinach

*The high chlorophyll sprouts such as snow pea and sunflower sprouts are highly recommended. Broccoli sprouts are very good for their anti-cancer properties.

Additional Ingredients:

To the foregoing ingredients feel free to add some raw seeds or nuts (best soaked for 6 hours – best nuts are almonds, walnut/pecan. Best seeds are pumpkin, hulled hempseeds, chia)

Some Examples of Healthy Dressings

Spirulina powder - 1 level teaspoonful of spirulina, 1 tablespoonful of flaxseed Oil or oil blend (such as Udo's Choice) 1 teaspoonful of cider vinegar, a pinch of Himalayan pink salt or sea-salt, black pepper (just mix together and serve as a dressing)

Vegan Avocado Mayo: This is a nice alternative to a lot of vegan mayonnaise products because it is made from fresh avocados or alternatively, cold-pressed avocado oil. It's simply made by blending together 1 large avocado, 1 crushed clove of garlic, juice of half a lemon, 1/3 of a cup of brine from chickpeas and a pinch of sea-salt I've also found one or two companies that sell it ready-made.

Coconut Aminos – a soya alternative that's derived from the sap of the coconut tree. It contains much less sodium than soya sauce. I use a brand called Coconut Secret which I like because of its flavour and pure composition.

Spicy Dressing - 1 tablespoonful of cider vinegar or lemon juice, 1 tablespoonful of flax or mixed oil blend, a pinch of sea-salt or Himalayan pink salt, crushed garlic, cayenne pepper, a dash of date syrup or brown rice syrup.

French Dressing – 3 tablespoonfuls of extra virgin olive oil, 1 tablespoonful of organic wine vinegar or cider vinegar, 1 teaspoon of French mustard, 1 teaspoon of date syrup, a pinch of sea-salt or Himalayan Pink salt and black pepper

Additional Salad Options

In order to vary your options, you can choose from the following salad recipes:

Green Salads

Green salads don't need to be boring lettuce leaf and tomato affairs. There are many different combinations and an equally wide variety of accompanying food ingredients that you can use. Leaves to choose from might include: Lettuce (all types), endive, chicory, spinach (including baby leaf), corn salad, watercress, cabbage, cress, etc. You can also add interesting flavours by using sprouted seeds, such as alfalfa, radish sprouts and fenugreek. Here is one example:

Serves 2-3

Green Leaf and Root Vegetable Salad

Serves 2-3

- 1-2 cups of shredded ice-burg lettuce
- 1 cup of alfalfa sprouts or sprouts of your choice
- ½ cup of finely chopped garden mint
- 1 cup of baby spinach
- 1 cup of corn salad (chopped)
- 1 medium sized red onion (finely chopped)
- 1 carrot (grated)
- 1 beetroot (grated)
- ½ cup of sunflower seeds

1. Place the leaves, sprouts and onions in a bowl and mix with your favourite dairy-free salad dressing, (e.g. French dressing)

2. Arrange the leaves in equal proportions on 2 or 3 plates and spread the grated carrots and beetroot over the top

3. Sprinkle with the sunflower seeds and drizzle with a little dressing

4. A good combination with baked butternut squash

Greek Tofu Salad

This is a good alternative to conventional Greek salad as it includes tofu as a substitute for feta cheese.

Serves 1

- 1 large green pepper (deseeded and sliced)
- 1 onion (peeled and sliced)
- 2 tomatoes (sliced)
- 50g of pitted black or green olives
- ½ cup of smoked or plain tofu chunks
- Oil and cider vinegar dressing (made with 1-part vinegar to 2 parts oil, sea salt, pepper and herbs).

1. Using a salad bowl, make layers of the slices of tomatoes, green peppers and onions

2. Add the olives and tofu pieces

3. Drizzle with the oil and vinegar dressing and serve

Apple, Sultana and Walnut Salad

Serves 1-2

- 2 eating apples (cored and sliced)
- Juice of one lemon
- 3 sticks of celery (chopped)
- 110g of walnut pieces

- 3 tbsp of vegan mayonnaise or plain almond yoghurt
- 3 tbsp of sultanas

1. Place the apples in a bowl and soak the slices in the lemon juice
2. Add the celery, sultanas and walnut pieces and mix well
3. Serve with the yoghurt or vegan mayonnaise dressing. Good with corn chips

Red Cabbage and Apple Salad

Serves 2

- 225g of red cabbage (shredded)
- 2 eating apples
- Juice of 1 lemon
- 1 tbsp of chopped chives
- 2 spring onions (finely chopped)
- 1 tsp of cumin seeds
- 2 tbsp of almonds (chopped)
- 1 tbsp of hazelnuts (chopped)
- 1tbsp of flaxseed oil
- Pinch of sea-salt
- Freshly ground black pepper

1. Remove the apple cores from the unpeeled apples. Grate and coat with lemon juice to prevent browning
2. Mix together the apples and shredded cabbage, spring onions. Sprinkle with the cumin seeds and oil. Season with the salt and pepper
3. Sprinkle with the almonds and hazelnuts and garnish with the chives
4. Serve with falafel or tofu chunks

Quinoa, Apricots and Avocado Salad

Serves 1-2

- 1 cup of quinoa
- 4 ready-soaked unsulphured apricots
- 200g of avocado (cubed)
- 2 tbsp of olive oil
- ¼ tsp of sea-salt

1. Simmer the quinoa in water for around 10-15 minutes until tender and all of the liquid has been absorbed
2. Drain the quinoa and place in a bowl with the apricots and seasoning
3. Stir the quinoa mixture ensuring all lumps are removed
4. Add the avocado cubes and oil and mix well
5. Serve

INFORMATION ON DRINKS AND SNACKS

Snacks

Fresh fruits, a small handful of unsalted raw nuts or seeds (pre-soaked if tolerated better); soaked dried organic fruits such as figs, dates or apricots soaked in a little almond yoghurt or coconut cream. A little raw chocolate.

Drinks

Herbal teas (make with pure filtered or spring water). Sweetened with a little date syrup or stevia if desired.

Dandelion coffee

Organic unsweetened fruit juice diluted 50:50 with pure water

Freshly made green juice, 2 sticks of celery, 1/3 of a cucumber, some green leaves – example, spinach or kale; 1 apple, ½ a lemon (unwaxed) and a piece of ginger

Nutri Bullet: Coconut water and spinach – makes a surprisingly creamy drink. Add a little green powder such as Dr Schulze for more nutrients

CHAPTER 9
Busting the Protein Myth

As most of us are aware, protein is needed by the body for a wide range of functions, including growth, repair of tissues, production of hormones and antibodies, etc. However, before reading this chapter, it might be useful to know that protein is made from a chain of building blocks known as amino acids. In fact, there are 20 total amino acids comprising of 9 essential amino acids and 11 non-essential amino acids. The essential ones are derived from our diet and the non-essential ones can be manufactured by the body.

9 Essential Amino Acids

Histidine	Isoleucine	Leucine	Lysine	Methionine

Phenylalanine	Threonine	Trytpophan	Valine

First of all, let's dispel some basic myths about protein consumption. These are some of the commonly held beliefs:

1. Protein deficiency is a real concern for vegans

2. A vegan diet makes you more at risk of developing a protein deficiency

3. Vegans have to pair plant proteins to get all of the amino acids to make a complete protein

If you adhere to a vegan diet and share some of these concerns, let me put your mind at rest.

Firstly, protein deficiency is very rare except for people who have severely restricted their diet; for example, with calorie restriction. Of course, elderly people are more at risk if they are not eating properly. Otherwise, as one might expect, people in countries where starvation exists are more likely to suffer from protein deficiency.

All Animals on Earth Rely on Plants

Secondly, almost all plant foods contain protein in varying amounts, which means that if you adhere to a vegan diet, providing that you get enough calories and consume a variety of different plant foods, then your protein requirements will be easily met. It's also worth bearing in mind that all the muscle-building amino acids come from plants. If it wasn't for plants there'd be no animals, including humans. Even carnivores like lions and wolves rely on plants because the animals that they prey on, such as buffalo and deer are built from plants.

Finally, current research indicates that we don't need to pair plant proteins to make a complete protein. Eating a variety of fruits, vegetables, whole grains and nuts/seeds, will ensure that we get more than enough protein to meet our requirements.

How Much Protein Does an Adult Require?

The requirements for protein are based upon your body weight. Adults should consume approximately 0.8 grams of protein per kilogram, or 2.2 pounds of body weight. Therefore, if you weigh 150 pounds or 68.2 kilograms, you need approximately 55 grams of protein per day.

This figure is arrived at by multiplying your weight in kilograms by 0.8. In this case:

68.2 x 0.8 = 54.56 or 55 grams in round figures.

Athletes may require slightly more protein per kilogram of body weight as intense activity results in the need for more muscle repair; however, we are talking here about 1.2 grams of protein per kilogram. Contrary to popular belief, protein supplements are usually not required as all protein needs should be met by food alone. This includes both vegan athletes and none athletes. The only caveat is that the daily caloric intake is adequate and that vegans consume a variety of plant- based foods, including a variety of fruits and vegetables, nuts/seeds, sprouted seeds, sea greens, pulses and whole grains.

The Dangers of having too Much Protein

"The major concern in terms of protein consumption comes from eating too much, rather than not enough. An excess of protein has been linked to a great number of health concerns".

Nutrition and Athletic Performance by Dr Douglas N. Graham

When I was a teenager, I took up the sport of weightlifting which took place in the YMCA in my home town of Sunderland (now a city) in north-east England. My involvement in weightlifting shifted towards bodybuilding, although I never entered in any bodybuilding competitions. During those early years I soon became aware of the emphasis upon getting enough protein; in fact, we were constantly being bombarded with adverts about protein drinks, protein bars, amino acid supplements and so forth. Not surprisingly, my fellow trainers jumped on the 'protein bandwagon'. They would consume copious amounts of brewer's yeast (high in protein and B vitamins), whey protein shakes, protein tablets and they made sure that they had plenty of animal proteins in their diet. Vegetable proteins were thought to be inferior. This kind of diet was considered essential if you wanted to build muscle. What's more, this was a message that was reinforced by the bodybuilding stars of the day; for example, Arnold Schwarzenegger, who believed that eating steak everyday helped to build muscle. If you listen to what he has to say about protein these days, it's good to hear that he's now in favour of a plant-based diet.

Now I did briefly adopt a high protein diet myself; however, I soon realised that it didn't make me feel good. In fact, my joints would usually become painful and I would feel generally unwell. This aroused my interest, so I began doing some research into the negative aspects of consuming too much protein and I soon learned that the consumption of excess protein can place a toxic load upon our liver and kidneys and make us very acidic, which in itself can lead to a variety of health issues including a weakened immune system.

So, now that I was a little more enlightened regarding the negative effects associated with consuming an excess of protein, I began to observe some of the other bodybuilders in my gym to see how they responded to this kind of high protein diet.

Interestingly enough, I noticed that a pattern was emerging. Basically, these bodybuilders would train well for a few weeks before coming down with some kind of illness; for example, influenza, a heavy cold or a gut infection. I also noticed that they would get injured more frequently. I soon concluded that the excess protein that they regularly consumed was leading to a high toxic load on their bodies and this in turn manifested itself in these health issues.

So, you might be asking, "What has all of this to do with my vegan diet?"

As I've already stated, the consumption of a wide variety of fruits and vegetables, including leafy greens, pulses and whole grains, adequately meets the needs of most people. If extra protein is needed for bodybuilders and athletes, this can be easily met by consuming raw nuts, seeds and protein-rich vegetables such as broccoli and spinach. You can also include the blue-green algae supplement, spirulina, which is approximately 60% easily assimilated protein. Compare this to beefsteak which contains around 22% protein. In addition, you can incorporate the likes of protein-rich powders such as pea protein, but remember to not overdo it for the reasons already stated.

In my own case, although in my sixties, I engage in weight training using quite heavy weights, including 100kg bench presses. I get all of my protein from fruits and vegetables, much to the amazement of my fellow trainers who consume animal proteins.

It's also interesting to note that a lot of world class athletes noticed a significant improvement in their performance when switching to a vegan diet. The film, **Game Changers (released on Netflix in 2019)** focuses upon a number of world class sportsmen and women who have made the change to a vegan diet with outstanding benefits to their health and sporting achievements. It features the likes of Formula One racing driver Lewis Hamilton, the world's number one male tennis player, Novak Djokovic and the aforementioned bodybuilder, Arnold Schwarzenegger. I highly recommend that you watch this incredibly inspiring film. The only caveat to this recommendation is that I feel the film doesn't focus enough on a healthy vegan diet, with its emphasis upon simply avoiding animal-based products such as meat, fish, dairy and eggs and not enough emphasis upon choosing the healthier vegan alternatives. I certainly subscribe to the view that by omitting these foods from the diet it will result in improved sporting performance and greater longevity; however, as you'll know by now if you've read the first part of this book, for long-term results I feel strongly that a vegan diet should be based upon whole foods and not processed foods.

Examples of Fruits and Vegetables Showing their Protein Content Per 100 grams

Vegetables

Asparagus:	2.2 grams	Cauliflower:	2.3 grams
Broccoli:	2.8 grams	Collards:	2.4 grams
Cabbage:	1.28 grams	Kale:	3.3 grams
Carrots:	0.93 grams	Spinach:	2.86 grams
Celery:	0.69 grams	Tomatoes:	0.88 grams

Fruits

Apples:	0.26 grams	Cantaloupe:	0.84 grams
Avocado:	2.00 grams	Grapes:	0.72 grams
Banana:	1.09 grams	Mango:	0.51 grams

Blackberry:	1.39 grams	Pineapple:	0.54 grams
Blueberry:	0.74 grams	Watermelon:	0.61 grams

Nuts/Seeds

Almonds:	21.22 grams	Macadamia:	7.91 grams
Brazil:	14.32 grams	Sesame:	17.73 grams
Cashews:	18.22 grams	Pine nuts:	13.69 grams
Coconut Meat:	3.33 grams	Hempseeds:	30.00 grams
Hazelnuts:	14.95 grams	Walnuts:	15.23 grams

Other Good Sources of Plant Proteins

Grains: Amaranth, buckwheat, brown rice, corn, millet, rye, teff and quinoa

Pulses: The protein content of most pulse legumes varies between 17-30%

Spirulina: This is a type of blue-green algae that has a high protein and vitamin content. In fact, 100 grams of spirulina provides an incredible 65 grams of protein, which is far higher than beef steak which contains around 22 grams per 100 grams of steak. This makes spirulina an excellent dietary addition for vegans.

Spirulina comes in various forms; namely, tablets, powder, sprinkles and flakes. I've also seen it in liquid form. When sourcing spirulina it's important to select a brand that is free from toxic contaminants (for example, heavy metals and pesticides). Therefore, it pays to do your home-work. One brand I like is called Gourmet Sprirulina, which is grown in India in a toxin-free environment. Moreover, this sprirulina is dried at a temperature of less than 42 degrees centigrade, so it retains its antioxidants, most notably phycocyanin, which gives spirulina it's blue-green colour.

Having said this, there are a number of good brands of spirulina available, but make sure that it's grown in a chemical-free environment and preferably not heated above 42 degree Centigrade.

CHAPTER 10
Key Nutrients for Vegans

As the food industry continues to make gains from the increasingly expanding vegan market with products such as vegan chips, meat substitutes such as burgers, sausages and desserts, it's important that vegans stay true to the key message embodied within this book; namely that care must be taken to ensure vegan food choices are still healthy ones. **Moreover, a vegan diet that is not well thought out may lead to nutritional deficiencies that can negatively impact upon health**

Aside from protein, which we've already discussed, vegans need to ensure that they have an adequate intake of the following essential nutrients:

Iron

Iron is an important component of haemoglobin which has the job of transporting oxygen to all parts of the body. It is essential for metabolism, normal cell function and growth. A lack of iron in the diet can result in anaemia and is characterised by symptoms that include breathlessness, hair loss and lack of energy.

Basically, there are two types of iron; haem and non-haem iron. The latter is from plant sources and the haem iron is from animal products. Vitamin C aids in the absorption of non-haem iron and since this form of iron is less easily absorbed, it's important to include in your diet iron and vitamin C rich foods such as citrus fruits, kiwi, capsicum and broccoli. Iron also comes from legumes, nuts and dark green leafy vegetables.

Calcium

Most people know that calcium is important for healthy bones and teeth, but did you know that it's also crucial for normal heart function, nervous signal transmission and muscle function?

Fortunately, we don't need to rely upon animal products such as dairy foods to supply us with enough of this important mineral. It can be derived from tofu, almonds, fortified soy and other plant milks in addition to dark green leafy vegetables such as spinach and collard greens.

Vitamin K

Vitamin K is required for proper blood clotting and bone health. Vegans who eat leafy greens on a regular basis should be getting adequate amounts of vitamin K, whilst those not getting enough may obtain an adequate supply from intestinal bacteria, unless these have been destroyed as a result of taking antibiotics.

Vitamin K refers to the chemical **menadione** and any derivatives of it that are important for blood clotting.

There are two types of vitamin K:

- Phylloquinone (K1) – found mostly in plant foods, especially in green leafy vegetables
- Menaquinone (K2) – found in animal tissues and also produced by bacteria. The only vegan food known to be high in K2 is **natto**, and vegan sources of supplemental K2 tend to be derived from this. Natto is made from soy beans fermented from a type of bacteria called **bacillus subtilis**

If you consume fermented foods and dark leafy greens on a regular basis, then it's unlikely that you'll need to supplement vitamin K; however, if you're following a vegan diet and don't consume these foods, then it's probably wise to take a supplemental form (K2) derived from natto.

Having said this, there's mounting evidence that when someone switches to a vegan diet, the increase in plant fibres helps to change the gut microbiome so that the vitamin K producing bacteria increase in numbers.

Good vegetable sources of vitamin K include: broccoli, kale, collards, spinach, Swiss chard, romaine lettuce and spirulina.

Omega-3 fatty acids

Omega-3 fatty acids, are an essential part of the membrane that surrounds our cells. They're also important for brain and heart health, reducing inflammation and numerous other bodily functions.

Plant sources of omega-3 fatty acids contain only alpha-linoleic acid (ALA) and are classed as being essential since our bodies cannot produce them. Once ingested, these fats are converted into eicosapentaenoic acid (EPA) and docosahexaenoic acid (DHA) which are ready to use by the body.

Good sources of ALA include flaxseeds, chia seeds and walnuts.

The problem that may arise for those following a vegan diet is that the amount of ALA that is converted from plant sources may not be that efficient.

Does this mean that vegans may not be getting enough EPA and DHA even if they consume plenty of ALA from plants? Well, if you're a good converter you'll probably be fine. However, if you're not, then you could end up with a deficiency.

Fortunately, over recent years, a solution has been found: a plant source of already converted EPA and DHA that comes from a marine alga called Schizochytrium. This is a supplement that provides a good source of DHA and EPA. These algae are usually grown in a controlled environment which has the advantage of the algae not being contaminated by marine pollution.

There's a number of supplement companies that sell this product and a quick search on Google will help you to source the best in your locality

Personally, in addition to supplementation, I also choose to include in my diet omega-rich foods such as flaxseeds, chia seeds and walnuts.

Caution: In his best-selling book, **Fats that Heal, Fats that Kill**, author and world-renowned expert on fats, **Udo Erasmus**, points out that due to the nutritional short-comings associated with a typical Western diet, most people are low in Omega 3 (ALA) essential fats and therefore usually benefit from including a good source of these in the diet; for example, flaxseed oil.

However, there is a caveat to his advice; namely, that exclusive reliance on this oil for all of our dietary needs can lead to an Omega 6 deficiency (Omega 6 essential fats work in tandem with Omega 3) after a year or so. He goes on to say that once any Omega 3 deficiency has been addressed, then it's important to switch to a more balanced oil blend that has a balance between Omega 3 and 6 essential fats. Basically, these fats are the ones that we need for health.I think this may have been the main driving force behind the formulation of Udo's oil blend, 'Udo's Choice', which is sold world-wide. There are also some other good oil blends on the market, but make sure the brand you select is stored in a stained-glass bottle to block light, and that it's been extracted without having been exposed to heat. Once opened, it should be kept air-tight and stored in the fridge.

Vitamin B12

Vitamin B12, also known as cobalamin, is a water-soluble vitamin involved in red blood cell production, DNA synthesis and brain health.

A deficiency in this key vitamin can cause serious health problems, including fatigue, digestive issues, nerve damage and neurological problems including depression and memory loss.

It's widely believed that B12 deficiency is a problem mostly associated with those following a vegetarian or vegan diet, since B12 is derived from animal sources including fish, meats, eggs and milk. However, studies have shown that B12 deficiency is widespread amongst those eating animal products. So why is this the case? Well, the simple answer is that if you're consuming animal products, you may be getting enough B12 from those sources, however, you may not be absorbing it very well. This is because B12 absorption is quite a complicated process that relies on a healthy and efficient digestive system. The problem is that many people's digestive systems are compromised by such factors as toxins, consumption of alcohol, infections, parasites (these are more common than most people realise), prescribed medications, antibiotics, consumption of processed foods and sensitivity to gluten (found in wheat, barley and rye as well as in many prepared ready meals). Even one of these factors can interfere with the absorption of this crucial vitamin. So, we can see that B12 deficiency isn't confined to vegans.

Interestingly, contrary to popular belief, animals don't make B12, since it's manufactured from bacteria that live in the soil and this is where animals get it from. For example, cattle from dirt that surrounds the grass and chickens when pecking for worms in the soil. Therefore, it stands to reason that when humans derive vitamin B12 as a result of eating animals or animal products, this vitamin is originally coming from the soil and is not being manufactured from the animal.

Since B12 is not available from eating plants, it's crucial that vegans either eat plenty of plant foods that are fortified with B12, and/or take a good quality B12 supplement. Personally, I wouldn't fully rely on fortified foods as a source. If you are a vegan, I would also suggest that you have regular blood tests to check your B12 level.

If you decide to take a B12 supplement, do remember that there are different forms of B12, namely, cyanocobalamin and methylcobalamin. Cyanocobalamin is the synthetic version and when it enters the body it's converted to either methylcobalamin or adenosylcobalamin which are the two natural active forms of B12 in humans. In my own case, I tend to opt for a supplement that contains the two natural forms in one tablet, thus avoiding a synthetic version of B12.

Vitamin D

Not too long ago it was believed that the most important function of vitamin D, along with calcium, is to maintain healthy bones and teeth and as protection from osteoporosis. We now know that it does so much more and that it's needed for reduction in inflammation and for immune and neuromuscular function. Although getting enough vitamin D is thought of as a vegan issue, it isn't really.

In fact, it's a much more generalised problem for those people who live in the northern hemisphere. So that includes countries such as the UK, Germany, Holland, northern France, Norway, Denmark, Greenland, Canada, New York, etc. The problem is a lack of year-round sunshine, since our bodies manufacture vitamin D as a result of exposure to sunlight; or to be precise, exposure to UVB rays, which make up one part of the light spectrum. In view of this, I believe that it's important that everyone living at these latitudes to supplement their diet with vitamin D. Having said this, vitamin D deficiency can even occur in people who live in hot climates if they're not getting enough sun exposure. For example, an office worker who spends most of their time working indoors.

Of course, we do get some vitamin D from certain foods, but unfortunately for vegans these foods are derived from animals such as cheese, fatty fish (like tuna and salmon) and egg yolks. Plant sources include mushrooms such as Portobello, maitake and shiitake varieties, in addition to fortified vegan milk such as coconut, almond and soya milks.

Vegans need to be aware that some vitamin D supplements are manufactured by irradiating sheep's wool, therefore, it's important to opt for a vitamin D supplement that is derived from plants, such as lichens.

Iodine

Iodine is another one of those vital nutrients that is often lacking in our modern diet. This is partly due to our over-farmed and artificially fertilised soils not providing enough of this mineral to meet the needs of growing crops, as well as other factors such as not eating as many seaweed products as we used to, and the increased use of chemicals called halogens which are present in our environment; for example, in flame retardants, drinking water and toothpaste.

These halogens are a family of elements on the periodic table that share similar chemical properties. Some of these can be toxic to your body; namely, fluorine (think fluoride found in some drinking water and most toothpastes), chlorine and bromine. Another halogen is that of iodine and this is the only halogen that the human body requires. The other three halogens, in addition to being toxic, tend to block your body's iodine receptors, thus preventing your cells from absorbing the iodine it needs to function normally.

This can be particularly detrimental to normal thyroid function, since iodine is needed by the thyroid in order to manufacture thyroid hormones such as thyroxine, a key function of which is to regulate the metabolic rate in the body. This is one reason why someone with an under-functioning thyroid (hypothyroidism) suffers from a slow metabolism and often feels excessively tired.

As with vitamin D deficiency, a lack of iodine is not exclusively a problem associated with a vegan diet, as it is widespread amongst the general population. However, vegans should ensure that they consume iodine-rich foods such as seaweed products (preferably sourced from relatively pollution-free areas) and prunes (5 dried prunes provide around 12 mcg of iodine, or about 9% of the daily value.

Iodine Supplements

A very good source of iodine is from a type of seaweed called kelp which can be taken as a tablet or in powder form.

Personally, I take 1-2 drops of a liquid iodine compound called Lugol's solution.

CAUTION! Anyone who suffers from a thyroid problem, for example hyperthyroidism, hypothyroidism, Hashimoto's or Grave's disease, should seek the advice of a qualified health professional before taking iodine supplements.

For further information I recommend that you read **Dr Brownstein's** book, **Iodine – Why You Need It, Why You Can't Live Without It**

I also suggest that you read **Lynne Farrow's** book:

The Iodine Crisis: What You Don't know about Iodine Can Wreck Your Life

Zinc

Zinc is another important nutrient that is crucial for normal growth and development. It's needed for synthesising protein, DNA development, wound healing and immune health.

A daily intake of zinc rich foods is essential as our bodies are unable to store it. Vegans can derive zinc by eating a variety of whole foods, including beans, seeds (for example pumpkin and sesame seeds), nuts (example, pine nuts, cashews and almonds) and whole grains. In addition, a good broad-spectrum multivitamin/mineral supplement should also contain zinc. I usually recommend a food state multi vitamin/mineral formula from a reputable company in preference to synthetic versions which form the basis of most supplements these days.

CHAPTER 11
Can a Healthy Vegan Diet Increase Longevity?

A number of scientific studies conducted around the world have revealed that the longest living people have certain lifestyle characteristics in common; namely, they live on a diet that is predominately plant based, featuring lots of fresh fruits and vegetables and very few, if any animal products.

Although their diets are not always entirely vegan, in most cases they're often close to it and their diet furnishes them with a wide range of nutrients, antioxidants, enzymes and natural health-promoting compounds such as anthocyanidins, carotenes quercetin and sulforaphane.

Consistent with the message that I've attempted to convey throughout this book, a number of these plant compounds have been shown to not only increase longevity, but also help to reduce the incidence of chronic diseases such as cardiovascular disease, cancer, neurological conditions and arthritis.

Unfortunately, many people residing in towns and cities with their fast food restaurants and supermarket convenience foods, don't adhere to these health-promoting dietary principles, and as a result they're prone to developing the so-called diseases of civilisation, in addition to suffering from the effects of premature ageing.

Contrast this with the fact that some of the longest living peoples of the world, such as the Hunza people from northern Pakistan, the natives of Vilcacamba in the southern region of Ecuador, the Abkhasia of the old Soviet Union, the Okinawans of Japan, the inhabitants of Sardinia in Italy, the Nicoya of Costa Rica and the Ikarians of Greece, all adhere to a similar type of lifestyle which include the following factors:

- Their diet consists of plenty of vegetables and fruits, mostly eaten in their raw state.

- Any grains that feature in the diet are unprocessed, containing all of the fibre and nutrients.

- They eat less overall

- They consume mostly healthy fats.

- They don't consume processed foods such as white sugar and other refined carbohydrates.

- They remain physically active throughout life (for example, the sheep herders of Sardinia who walk an average for at least 5 miles per day). Moreover, their diet furnishes them with the right nutrients needed to optimise their health and mobility; in other words, there is a lack of arthritis and other conditions that impact adversely on mobility.

- They adopt a positive attitude towards life and ageing.

Obviously, in terms of diet, there are some regionally influenced differences; for example, the Okinawans include some soya in their diet. Nevertheless, it is clear that such a natural diet would result in a low level of toxins in the body and a high level of vitamins, minerals, enzymes and antioxidants. All of these factors make for a potent influence on the ageing process. If we were to compare the internal environment of let's say, the average Okinawan, to that of an average adult from somewhere such as New York or London, I believe that the differences in toxicity levels would speak for themselves. For a start, people who live in highly populated cities are exposed to more environmental pollution, such as exhaust fumes. Their water supply is often laced with toxic substances such as fluoride, nitrates, heavy metals, hormones and chlorine, and their food is far more likely to be of a highly processed nature, high in saturated and hydrogenated fats, salt, refined carbohydrates, numerous chemical additives and pesticides. Add to this the vast array of chemicals in packaging, cosmetics and household cleaning materials to which most of us are exposed, and we begin to get the picture.

Again, if we compare the aforementioned peoples in contrast to their city dwelling counterparts, it is known that they have a very low incidence of cancer, heart disease, diabetes, high blood pressure, strokes, Alzheimer's disease, etc. Now, the significant thing here is that all of these diseases are much more prevalent with the onset of advancing years. So, again, the question we must ask is: why do the likes of the Abkhasians and Vilcabambans have such a low incidence of the so-called degenerative diseases? The answer, in my view and that of an increasing number of scientists, is the powerful combination of a very healthy diet and low exposure to pollution.

 This view is certainly reinforced when we consider the case of the 1,500 monks who live on Mount Athos in northern Greece. In recent times they have been the subject of studies because of their astonishingly low rates of cancer. In fact, since 1994 the monks have been regularly tested and only eleven of them have developed prostate cancer – a disease commonly associated with advancing age in men. Incredibly, one study revealed that their rate of lung and bladder cancer was zero.

Apparently, life on Athos has changed very little over the last 1,043 years. A typical day begins with a simple breakfast consisting of hard bread and tea; whilst much of the monks' day is taken up with chores such as cooking, cleaning and attending to crops. The final meal of the day consists of the likes of lentils, salad and fruits. Haris Aidonopoulis, a urologist at the University of Thessalonika, has this to say about the monks' diet, which involves them avoiding olive oil, wine and dairy produce on Mondays, Wednesdays and Fridays:

"What seems to be the key, it's not only what we call the Mediterranean diet, but also eating the old-fashioned way. Small simple meals at regular intervals are very important."

In addition to eating little dairy foods, the monks do not eat meat, preferring fish. The avoidance of dairy products, wine and olive oil for three days per week helps to eke out their food supplies. In terms of life expectancy, this could be significant, as dietician Michalis Hourdakis from Athens University explains:

"This limited consumption of calories has been found to lengthen life. Meat has been associated with intestinal cancer, while fruit and vegetables help ward off prostate cancer."

No doubt the lack of air pollution on Mount Athos, in addition to the monks' active lifestyle also plays its part in the monk's longevity and low incidence of cancer.

Now, before you throw your hands in the air exclaiming: "So if I want to live a long and youthful life I have to live like a monk!" let me reassure you that this isn't the message that I'm trying to convey here. What I am saying, is that there are certain principles inherent in the diet and lifestyle of these monks, which are consistent with the lifestyles of several long-lived peoples around the world who live on a diet of natural unprocessed foods.

The question is: **can we do even better by omitting those animal products and living exclusively on a vegan whole foods diet?** Personally, I firmly believe this to be true and it's a view shared by the Director of The Hippocrates Health Institute, **Brian Clement, Ph.D., L.N.**

The HHI is based in Florida and set in several acres of tropical gardens. It's a place where people with a variety of health challenges can go in order to engage in the 3-week Life-Change Programme. A key component of the program is the diet, which consists of a 80% raw and 20% cooked food vegan diet. Ideally, they want you to be 100% raw and the initial 20% cooked food is to help people to make the transition to an entirely raw vegan diet. People who have followed the programme and then continued with the diet when they return home, have achieved some significant improvements in their health, including reversal of some serious chronic health conditions.

Brian Clement is of the firm opinion that avoiding all animal products is a major factor when it comes to working with the body's innate healing abilities and promoting longevity.

The following statement, from which I quote from their website, sums up their philosophy:

"With hundreds of thousands of people participating in this program over the last half century, volumes of data have been accrued, giving Clement a privileged insight into the lifestyle required to prevent disease, enhance longevity, and maintain vitality and stamina."

So, there we have it; yet more evidence that supports the conclusion that a vegan whole foods lifestyle is the most conducive towards good health and extending an active life.

CHAPTER 12
Avoiding the Toxic Trap

Detoxification – How to tackle internal pollution using organically-grown fruits and vegetables and one of nature's most remarkable minerals

It's a sobering thought but the world is becoming increasingly toxic, and as a result, so are we humans. What's more, it's no longer the case that the greatest source of toxins is concentrated around the most developed and densely populated areas, such as the big cities and industrial complexes. How do we know? Well, consider the Arctic region. We tend to think that its distance from industrialised countries ensures that it is relatively clean and pollution free. However, this couldn't be further from the truth, since the Arctic is on the receiving end of contaminants generated from thousands of miles away. In fact, in recent years, scientists have discovered a broad range of toxic substances in the region. These include pesticides, radioactivity from Chernobyl and heavy metals such as mercury, a by-product from various industrial processes.

Nor does it end there, since it appears that the Arctic is also a collection area for much of the world's air pollution; including smoke and particulates from forest fires from northern Europe, North America and Asia.

So, the point I'm making here is that pollution doesn't recognize boundaries. This is blindingly obvious when we consider how the Chernobyl nuclear explosion produced fall-out that contaminated large areas of Europe, including the UK, where radioactive hotspots over mountainous regions in parts of Wales and the Scottish Highlands still exist. This is why, for example, sheep from certain hill farms in Wales are still monitored for radioactivity. Moreover, in 2011, we had the Fukishima disaster when a giant tsunami severely damaged nuclear plants in Japan resulting in massive fall-out, which continues to this day.

Well, so much for the global environment; what about our internal environment? It obviously stands to reason that our bodies are the recipients of toxins that we are subjected to via the air we breathe, the water we drink and of course, the food we eat. And what about all of those chemicals with the unpronounceable names that are lurking in everyday household detergents, cosmetics and even in the very fabric of the buildings that we spend most of our lives in? The fact is, we humans are being subjected to toxins that didn't even exist not that long ago. If you're not entirely convinced, just consider this sample of contaminants that we're exposed to on a daily basis:

Heavy metals such as lead, mercury, aluminium and cadmium; pesticides, artificial fertilisers, fungicides, herbicides, chlorine and flouride (from tap water and toothpaste), benzene and hydrocarbons (from vehicle exhausts); PCB's (polychlorinated biphenyls from plastics and other sources), dioxins (formed as a result of combustion processes), phthalates (used to lengthen the life of fragrances and soft plastics), radioactive contaminants such as strontium 90 and caesium 137 and a wide range of additives in processed foods.

Pesticides

"We put poison on our crops and we then eat the poison!"

I recently came across this profound statement about agricultural chemicals and I must admit I can't recall the source. However, for me it really sums up the insanity.

Fortunately, an increasing number of people around the world are becoming aware of the potential dangers associated with long-term exposure to agricultural chemicals, including pesticides. There are organisations in different countries that are trying to promote safe alternatives. For example, in the UK we have the **Pesticide Action Network UK (PAN UK)**. On their Home Page they make the following statement:

We are the only UK charity focused on tackling the problems caused by pesticides and promoting safe and sustainable alternatives in agriculture, urban areas, homes and gardens.

I highly recommend that you visit their website which contains a wide range of valuable information on the dangers associated with pesticide use on our crops. They also include a lot of research on the adverse effects of pesticides on humans, animals and the environment.

www.pan-uk.org/

In order to assess the level of pesticides used on fruits and vegetables, each year the UK government conducts tests on a range of produce. Using data over a 5-year period, PAN have formulated a list that they refer to as the 'dirtiest' and 'cleanest' fruits and vegetables based on how many of the samples tested revealed residues of more than one pesticide. They decided to focus upon multiple residues due to the current regulatory system which is designed to assess the safety of one pesticide at a time, which doesn't take into account the so-called "cocktail effect", when interactions between different pesticides may have more potent adverse effects upon living organisms.

PAN UK kindly gave me permission to use the following illustration regarding their list of the most contaminated fruits and vegetables compared to the ones found to contain the least residues:

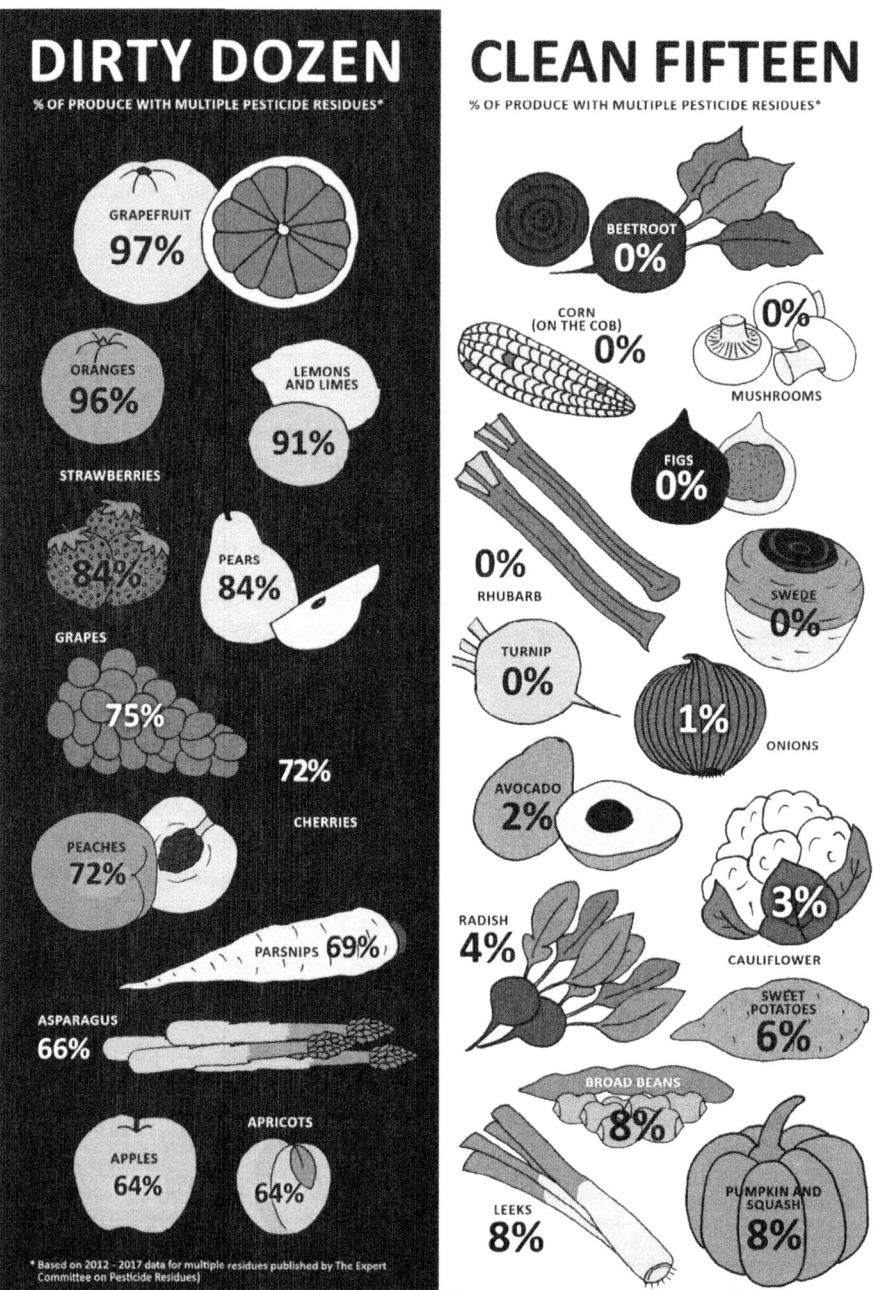

DIRTY DOZEN
% OF PRODUCE WITH MULTIPLE PESTICIDE RESIDUES*

GRAPEFRUIT
97%

ORANGES
96%

LEMONS AND LIMES
91%

STRAWBERRIES
84%

PEARS
84%

GRAPES
75%

72%
CHERRIES

PEACHES
72%

PARSNIPS **69%**

ASPARAGUS
66%

APRICOTS

APPLES
64%

64%

* Based on 2012 – 2017 data for multiple residues published by The Expert Committee on Pesticide Residues)

CLEAN FIFTEEN
% OF PRODUCE WITH MULTIPLE PESTICIDE RESIDUES*

BEETROOT
0%

CORN (ON THE COB)
0%

0%
MUSHROOMS

FIGS
0%

0%
RHUBARB

SWEDE
0%

TURNIP
0%

1%
ONIONS

AVOCADO
2%

3%
CAULIFLOWER

RADISH
4%

SWEET POTATOES
6%

BROAD BEANS
8%

LEEKS
8%

PUMPKIN AND SQUASH
8%

The 'Cocktail' Effect

In my opinion, the everyday use of agricultural chemicals on our food crops represents a major experiment on the human race. None of the so-called experts on pesticides can prove that exposure to a single pesticide is safe, let alone exposure to several different pesticides, along with herbicides, fungicides and artificial nitrates.

Vulnerable Groups

Are certain groups within society more vulnerable to the effects of pesticides?

PAN UK has this to say on the subject:

Certain groups of people are more susceptible to the effects of pesticides, especially young children and expectant mothers. Exposure to certain pesticides at critical stages in development can interfere with particular organs and their functions. Of particular concern are endocrine disrupting chemicals which affect hormone systems in the body and have been associated with learning disabilities, attention deficit disorder, and cognitive and brain development problems

Overall, these contaminants are frequently thought to be associated with causing diseases such as various cancers, neurological illnesses (such as Alzheimer's disease), arthritis, M.E., chronic fatigue syndrome and premature ageing.

Of course, most people these days are aware that we should be eating healthier in order to increase our resistance to illness. However, unfortunately, this isn't always enough

Is your diet acting as a slow poison?

It's often said that you are what you eat. As a population we're getting sicker and sicker, which is why we should turn to our diet to correct what is out of balance, and bring in plenty of healing foods, such as organic fruits and vegetables. Generally speaking, if you're adhering to a vegan diet then it's likely that you'll be automatically omitting some key sources of toxins found in animal produce; for example, chicken and beef from animals that have been reared in factory farms; fish from polluted seas and oceans and milk from cow's fed on grains tainted with agricultural chemicals. Having said this, as already highlighted in this chapter, being a vegan or following a predominately plant-based diet does not mean that we are immune from exposure to the pervasive poisons that are in the food we eat, the water we drink and the very air that we breathe.

Toxins Overwhelm the Immune System

Despite what most medical practitioners say to the contrary, our bodies have not evolved to fight the magnitude of this toxic attack, and we simply can't rid ourselves of toxins fast enough, which causes them to be stored mainly in our fat cells and tissues. Much like a dripping tap eventually fills up the sink and floods, this everyday exposure builds up over time, until it overwhelms our immune system.

Perhaps it's no coincidence that the symptoms of low-dose chronic toxic exposure look a lot like what many people just write off as being related to getting older:

- Feeling tired, with low energy levels
- Difficulty sleeping or insomnia
- Headaches or migraines
- Often catching colds or vulnerability to infections
- Impaired digestion or feeling bloated
- Weight gain, especially around the belly area
- Aching muscles and joints

This is not normal! Or at least, it doesn't have to be.

Zeolites – A Cornerstone of Detoxification

Increasingly, detoxification is recognised as not just an option but a necessity. Your choices include juicing leafy green vegetables, sweating it out in conventional saunas and far infra-red saunas, or even colonics (for the brave of heart).

While each method has its merits, none can truly systemically detoxify the body of heavy metals and toxins. All of which is why zeolites, or specifically, the zeolite Clinoptilolite, is getting a lot of attention these days. This natural mineral possesses unique qualities that allow it to selectively bind with toxins, taking out the bad and leaving in the good.

A Crystalline Structure that Traps Toxins

Zeolites are crystals formed when volcanic molten lava meets the sea, and this chemical reaction creates a crystal with a cage-like, porous structure and negative charge, making it one of the rare, negatively-charged minerals in nature.

This negative charge is what makes it a natural detoxifier, since most environmental toxins and heavy metals carry a positive charge; and opposites attract! Clinoptilolite has an affinity for mercury, lead, cadmium, aluminium and even volatile organic compounds found in paint and plastics.

Granted GRAS (generally recognised as safe) status by the Food & Drug Administration, this natural mineral is completely safe, and leaves the body within 4-6 hours. Now, you'll find zeolite readily available, but as I discovered, there are three things you should look for before buying a zeolite supplement.

Three Questions You Have to Ask:

What size are the zeolite particles?

Off the shelf, zeolites can range from 10 to 40 microns in size, which will only detox your colon and not your cells. To get into the bloodstream, the particles have to be reduced in size so they are 0.5 microns or smaller. That's about 100 times smaller than the width of a human hair. Check to make sure the provider includes a particle size test to verify what you're getting.

What type of zeolite is it?

There are many kinds of zeolite. Since Clinoptilolite has well-established safety studies, and peer-reviewed research, you'll want to make sure that's what you're getting. The provider should do x-ray diffraction analysis to confirm a high percentage of Clinoptilolite.

Has the zeolite been cleaned?

In nature, zeolites do what they were made to do (attract toxins) which means that any mined zeolite can be full of lead, arsenic and other environmental toxins. Inside the zeolite, they're unlikely to do harm but will render it ineffective as the zeolite is too full to trap any toxins from the body. So, ask for an independent certificate of analysis.

What Can You Expect?

When sized for absorption and properly prepared, there's no denying the power of Clinoptilolite to attract and remove heavy metals and environmental toxins, safely and effectively, which is why this zeolite should be part of your lifestyle.

During an initial detox, feelings of tiredness can occur, so hydrate well with pure water. As heavy metals and toxins begin to leave the body (inside the zeolite), your systems come back into balance and you can expect improvements in sleep quality, energy levels, mental clarity, and enhanced immune response, possibly making this one mineral a perfect antidote to the poisons we face every day. And remember, just because you may be following a vegan diet and lifestyle, doesn't mean to say that you're not ingesting toxins on a daily basis, especially if you're consuming a lot of conventionally-grown produce.

Acknowledgement

I would like to thank Touchstone Essentials for their input in providing information on zeolite, particularly because they have much expertise and the highest standards in terms of producing quality zeolite products.

They have kindly provided the following scientific information on clinoptilolite (the most active form of zeolite).

If you require further information on sourcing reputable brands or purchasing zeolite please contact me via my email address: bio_cure@ hotmail.com

Alternatively, you can visit Touchstone Essentials at:

Pure Body: https://thegoodinside.com/shop/product/pure-body/

Lab Analysis: https://thegoodinside.com/wp-content/uploads/PB_ LabAnalysis_Oct2018.pdf ·

Particle Size: https://thegoodinside.com/wp-content/uploads/ PureBody_Particle_Size_10_18.pdf

X-Ray Diffraction: https://assets.thegoodinside.com/wp-content/ uploads/PureBody_Particle_Size_10_18.pdf

Summary

My principle objective in writing this book was to not only highlight the dangers associated with the regular consumption of vegan processed foods, but to also empower the reader with information about the lifestyle choices that can potentially result in good health and a long and useful life, both of which, I think you'll agree, are truly worthwhile aims.

So, if you've decided to opt for a whole food vegan lifestyle, congratulations! You'll not only be living in harmony with the planet on which we all co-exist, but it's my express belief, and one that I hope you'll come to share, that working with the natural laws (nature), will reward you with the priceless gift of good health.

To help you on your journey I've summarised the following key principles that are embodied within this book:

Try to avoid or at least minimise your consumption of processed plant foods, Including all oils, refined grains, sugars, additives, etc.

Aim to base your diet on a variety of vegetables, fruits, sprouted seeds, whole grains, sea-greens, nuts and seeds.

Don't overdo the fats. A lot of people give up eating animal products and in switching to a vegan diet begin eating lots of nuts, seeds and avocadoes. They also often use a lot of oils in their meal preparation.

This results in low energy and overall poor health. Therefore, it's best to avoid using these foods as a main ingredient in your recipes. Use them as condiments instead; for example, salad dressing made with flaxseed oil

Ensure that you're not risking nutrient deficiencies by using good quality supplements, preferably food state rather than synthetic. Vitamins B12 and D along with omega 3 and 6 essential fats are especially important.

Follow the 80:20 diet rule to ensure that your system is alkaline and not too acidic

Try to implement a periodic detox such as my 7 Day Alkaline diet and try to opt for organically-grown produce whenever possible.

Useful Information

References: Chapter 7

(1) https://www.ncbi.nlm.nih.gov/pubmed/19476292

(2) Molecules. 2019 Sep 13;24(18). pii: E3335. doi: 10.3390/molecules24183335.

Apple Peel Flavonoid Fraction 4 Suppresses Breast Cancer Cell Growth by Cytostatic and Cytotoxic Mechanisms

Loung CY[1], Fernando W[2], Rupasinghe HPV[3],[4], Hoskin DW

(3) https://www.greenmedinfo.com/article/apples-contain-compounds-which-induce-programmed-cell-death-human-stomach-cancer

(4) https://www.ncbi.nlm.nih.gov/pubmed/28196336

(5) https://www.ncbi.nlm.nih.gov/pubmed

(6) Effect of increased potassium intake on cardiovascular risk factors and disease: systematic review and meta-analyses.

Aburto NJ[1], Hanson S, Gutierrez H, Hooper L, Elliott P, Cappuccio FP

(7) https://www.ncbi.nlm.nih.gov/pubmed/1308699

(8) https://pubmed.ncbi.nlm.nih.gov/15455348

Fruits, vegetables and risk of renal cell carcinoma: a prospective study of Swedish women.

Rashidkhani B[1], Lindblad P, Wolk A.

(9) https://www.greenmedinfo.com/article/beetroot-juice-supplementation-may-be-effective-performance-improvement-during high intensity exercise

(10) Radioprotective activity of betalains from red beets in mice exposed to gamma irradiation

Eur J Pharmacol. 2009 Aug 1;615(1-3):223-7. Epub 2009 May 14.
PMID: 19446548

(11) https://www.greenmedinfo.com/search/google-cse#gsc.q=beets and prostate cancer

(12) https://www.ncbi.nlm.nih.gov/pmc/articles/PMC2862148

(13) https://www.ncbi.nlm.nih.gov/pubmed/24997566

(14) https://www.ncbi.nlm.nih.gov/pubmed/23319811

(15) https://www.ncbi.nlm.nih.gov/pubmed/31123866

(16) https://www.ncbi.nlm.nih.gov/pubmed/18163565

(17) https://www.ncbi.nlm.nih.gov/pmc/articles/PMC1643665

(18) https://link.springer.com/article/10.1007/s40495-014-0002-x

(19) https://www.ncbi.nlm.nih.gov/pmc/articles/PMC2782876

(20) https://www.ncbi.nlm.nih.gov/pmc/articles/PMC3042791

(21) https://www.ncbi.nlm.nih.gov/pubmed/23440782

(22) https://www.ncbi.nlm.nih.gov/pubmed/18454549

(23) https://www.ncbi.nlm.nih.gov/pmc/articles/PMC3550877

(24) https://www.ncbi.nlm.nih.gov/pubmed/14973107

(25) https://www.ncbi.nlm.nih.gov/pubmed/14569406

(26) https://www.ncbi.nlm.nih.gov/pubmed/16908818

(27) https://www.ncbi.nlm.nih.gov/pubmed/23679237

(28) https://www.ncbi.nlm.nih.gov/pmc/articles/PMC4637098

(29) https://www.ncbi.nlm.nih.gov/pmc/articles/PMC3870206

(30) https://www.ncbi.nlm.nih.gov/pubmed/15670984

(31) https://www.ncbi.nlm.nih.gov/pubmed/17301257

(32) https://www.ncbi.nlm.nih.gov/pubmed/24869971

(33) https://www.ncbi.nlm.nih.gov/pubmed/25163498

(34) https://www.ncbi.nlm.nih.gov/pubmed/11697022

(35) https://pubmed.ncbi.nlm.nih.gov/20594781-aged-garlic-extract-lowers-blood-pressure-in-patients-with-treated-but-uncontrolled-hypertension-a-randomised-controlled-trial

(36) https://pubmed.ncbi.nlm.nih.gov/24035939-effects-of-allium-sativum-garlic-on-systolic-and-diastolic-blood-pressure-in-patients-with-essential-hypertension

(37) https://pubmed.ncbi.nlm.nih.gov/8169881-garlic-as-a-lipid-lowering-agent-a-meta-analysis

(38) https://pubmed.ncbi.nlm.nih.gov/16484570-garlic-reduces-dementia-and-heart-disease-risk

(39) https://www.ncbi.nlm.nih.gov/pmc/articles/PMC4103721

(40) https://draxe.com/health/blue-zones

(41) https://pubmed.ncbi.nlm.nih.gov/26800498-grapes-vitis-vinifera-as-a-potential-candidate-for-the-therapy-of-the-metabolic-syndrome

(42) https://pubmed.ncbi.nlm.nih.gov/23517616-the-anti-inflammatory-potential-of-phenolic-compounds-in-grape-juice-concentrate-g8000tm-on-246-trinitrobenzene-sulphonic-acid-induced-colitis

(43) https://www.ncbi.nlm.nih.gov/pmc/articles/PMC3916869

(44) https://pubmed.ncbi.nlm.nih.gov/11412050-the-effect-of-fruit-and-vegetable-intake-on-risk-for-coronary-heart-disease

(45) https://www.sciencedirect.com/science/article/pii/S0271531705801757

(46) https://www.ncbi.nlm.nih.gov/pmc/articles/PMC2581754

(47) https://pubmed.ncbi.nlm.nih.gov/18290732-quantitative-assessment-of-citric-acid-in-lemon-juice-lime-juice-and-commercially-available-fruit-juice-products

(48) https://onlinelibrary.wiley.com/doi/full/10.1111/j.1541-4337.2008.00047.x

(49) https://pubmed.ncbi.nlm.nih.gov/28181586-protective-effect-of-mangiferin-on-myocardial-ischemia-reperfusion-injury-in-streptozotocin-induced-diabetic-rats-role-of-age-ragemapk-pathways

(50) https://pubmed.ncbi.nlm.nih.gov/25866155-consuming-lentinula-edodes-shiitake-mushrooms-daily-improves-human-immunity-a-randomized-dietary-intervention-in-healthy-young-adults

(51) https://www.sciencedirect.com/topics/immunology-and-microbiology/lentinan

(52) https://www.ncbi.nlm.nih.gov/pmc/articles/PMC1160565

(53) https://pubmed.ncbi.nlm.nih.gov/25070597-medicinal-properties-of-hericium-erinaceus-and-its-potential-to-formulate-novel-mushroom-based-pharmaceuticals

(54) https://pubmed.ncbi.nlm.nih.gov/24266378-neurotrophic-properties-of-the-lions-mane-medicinal-mushroom-hericium-erinaceus-higher-basidiomycetes-from-malaysia

(55) https://pubmed.ncbi.nlm.nih.gov/21068346-hesperidin-contributes-to-the-vascular-protective-effects-of-orange-juice-a-randomized-crossover-study-in-healthy-volunteers

(56) https://pubmed.ncbi.nlm.nih.gov/23859487-both-red-and-blond-orange-juice-intake-decreases-the-procoagulant-activity-of-whole-blood-in-healthy-volunteers

(57) https://www.zora.uzh.ch/id/eprint/45805

(58) https://link.springer.com/article/10.1007/s11130-013-0343-3

(59) https://pubmed.ncbi.nlm.nih.gov/6912244

(60) https://pubmed.ncbi.nlm.nih.gov/25505983

(61) https://pubmed.ncbi.nlm.nih.gov/28065968

(62) https://pubmed.ncbi.nlm.nih.gov/22191568

(63) https://pubmed.ncbi.nlm.nih.gov/26992121

(64) https://pubmed.ncbi.nlm.nih.gov/21409897

(65) https://pubmed.ncbi.nlm.nih.gov/26992121

(66) https://pubmed.ncbi.nlm.nih.gov/17906180

(67) https://pubmed.ncbi.nlm.nih.gov/28846633

(68) https://www.ncbi.nlm.nih.gov/pmc/articles/PMC3068482

(69) https://pubmed.ncbi.nlm.nih.gov/22158914

(70) https://pubmed.ncbi.nlm.nih.gov/10050865

(71) https://pubmed.ncbi.nlm.nih.gov/12010859

(72) https://pubmed.ncbi.nlm.nih.gov/16465309

(73) https://pubmed.ncbi.nlm.nih.gov/17352962

(74) https://www.ncbi.nlm.nih.gov/pmc/articles/PMC4464475/?X

(75) https://www.ncbi.nlm.nih.gov/pmc/articles/PMC4464475

ORGANISATIONS

Pesticide Action Network UK
https://www.pan-uk.org/

The Gerson Institute: Uses a natural plant-based diet and juicing to help restore health in individuals with challenging health conditions
https://gerson.org/gerpress/

The Hippocrates Health Institute, West Palm Beach, Florida: Uses a raw living foods, plant-based diet and green juices to help people with challenging illnesses to restore health

The Organic Consumer's Association
https://www.organicconsumers.org/

The Soil Association UK
https://www.soilassociation.org/our-standards/what-are-organic-standards/

The Vegan Society
https://www.vegansociety.com/

RECOMMENDED COMPANIES

USA sprout company: ISS (International Specialty Supply)
info@sproutnet.com
https://sproutnet.com

International Sprout Grower's Association
https://isga-sprouts.org/about-sprouts/sprout-history/

Gourmet Spirulina
Email: hello@gourmet-spirulina.co.uk

Clean Machine vegan supplements were designed by vegan bodybuilder Geoff Palmer who wanted to offer supplements that contained the best ingredients to support health and fitness. His products are a welcome change from most of the protein and other supplements that contain artificial ingredients, etc.
https://cleanmachineonline.com/

Vegus Juices: Producers of high quality cold pressed juices including wheatgrass and broccoli sprouts juice
https://vegusjuices.com/tag/raw/

Touchstone Essentials: Produce good quality zeolite products and other health-promoting products
https://thegoodinside.com/

A.Vogel: Herbal company founded by famous Swiss herbalist Alfred Vogel
https://www.avogel.co.uk/avogel-world/

Coconut Flat Bread
As I'm a great advocate of using plant-based foods that use only healthy ingredients, I was excited to sample some delicious coconut bread from a company in the UK called Calvin's Free From Foods. They use the finest organic ingredients and no additives whatsoever and it's so refreshing to come across a company that actually care about the health of their customers. You can get more information here: http://calvinsfreefromfoods.co.uk/

Scalarwave Laser

The Scalarwave Laser is an approved over-the-counter medical device. The laser is very beneficial for pain relief, relaxation of tissue, increase circulation, decrease inflammation and arthritis. The laser is a wellness tool that supports the body's ability to achieve and maintain homeostasis.

www.ilovemylaser.com

Contact: Lucretia
Telephone: +1 001 424 653 9587 (USA)

Far infra-red Appliances

Far infrared home and clinic appliances using advanced low EMF emission technology that helps with challenging conditions such as arthritis, circulatory problems, stress and detoxification.

https://www.get-fitt.com/far_infrared_treatment_for_arthritis/fibromyalgia/

Rife Machine

In my experience Rife machines can be very expensive and cost prohibitive for many people. I was therefore, pleased to come across what turned out to be an ethical company that aimed to provide a Rife machine designed to not only support the user's health, but also a machine that was around a fifth of the price of comparable machines on the market, thus making it more accessible to many.

For Contact and Inquiries:
Rosalie at: www.rifedigital.net
Direct Email: rifedigitaluk@gmail.com
Telephone: 0044 (0)7376056374

BOOKS

A Life in Healing by Jan de Vries; Mainstream Publishing

Crazy, Sexy Diet, by Kris Carr; Skirt Books

Cancer Medicine from Nature: The Herbal Cancer Formulas of Edgar Cayce & Harry Hoxsey by Roger Bloom; Eco Images Publishing (Second Edition)

Grain Damage: Rethinking the High-Starch Diet, by Douglas N. Graham

80-10-10 Diet: Balancing Your Health, Your Weight and Your Life – One Luscious Bite at A Time, By Douglas N. Graham

Fats That Heal Fats that Kill by Udo Erasmus; Alive Books

Iodine - Why You Need It, Why You Can't Live Without it: Dr David Brownstein www.drbrownstein.com

Living Foods for Optimal Health by Brian R Clement; Prima Publishing

Optimum Nutrition For Vegans: How to be healthy and optimally nourished on a plant-based diet by Patrick Holford; Piatkus Books

The Hippocrates Diet and Health Program (Natural Diet and Health Program for Weight Control; Disease) by Anne Wigmore and Dennis Weaver

The Raw Cure: Healing Beyond Medicine by Jesse J Jacoby; Soulspire Publishing

The Beginner's Guide to a Plant-Based Diet by Brandon Hearn; printed in Great Britain by Amazon

The Sprouter's Handbook by Edward Cairney; Argyll Publishing

The Nature Doctor by Alfred Vogel; Mainstream Publishing

The Wheatgrass Book by Anne Wigmore; Avery (a member of the Penguin Group) (USA)

Super Juiced me! 28 Day Juice Plan by Jason Vale; Juice Master Publications

Printed in Great Britain
by Amazon

53448469R00086